WORLD-CLASS HEALTH CARE

HOSPITALS AND MEDICAL COLLEGES

Five Pillars: AI, Digital Transformation, Quality, Leadership, and Humanity

By

JAY P. PATEL

Published by

OWL® PUBLISHERS

www.owlpublishers.com

360 S Market St, San Jose, CA 95113,

United States.

Printed in the United States of America

This book is dedicated to

My parents & Thol Village

farmers from the village of Thol, Gujarat,

who taught me by their lives that hard work, love, family, and education

can transform what is possible for a person, a family, and a community.

To every patient-----

who deserve world-class care regardless of where they were born,

how much they earn, or what language they speak.

You are the reason this book exists.

To every healthcare leader, educator, and student

who carries the conviction that excellence is achievable,

that transformation is always possible,

and that the patient must always remain at the center.

And to the vision & dream of Bhagyoday

a new dawn, rising for the community of Kadi, Gujarat,

Jay P. Patel

FOREWORD

By Dr. Shrenik Shah, board-certified Vascular and Interventional Radiologist

When a Book Finds You at the Right Moment

There are books you read for knowledge. There are books you read for professional development. And then, rarely, there are books that seem to articulate, with clarity and conviction, something you have known in your bones for years but could never quite organize into words. This is one of those books.

I have spent my career at the intersection of radiology and surgery, two disciplines that demand precision above all else. Every image I read is a question with a life-changing answer. Every procedure is a moment of irreversible action. In this world, error is not abstract, and excellence is not aspirational; it is moral.

When Jay Patel asked me to review this book and provide the Foreword, I expected a thoughtful book about artificial intelligence in healthcare. What I found was something more ambitious, more grounded, and more urgently needed: a blueprint for how healthcare & education must change, how its people must be trained, how its systems must be built, and how its values must be protected as technology reshapes everything around us.

The View From Radiology: Where AI Arrived First

If you want to understand what AI & digital Transformation can do in healthcare, and what it cannot do, ask a radiologist. Our specialty was the first to feel the full force of this transformation. AI-powered image analysis arrived in our reading rooms years before it reached most other clinical disciplines, and with it came every question this book addresses: Does AI replace the physician? Does it enhance judgment or erode it? How do you validate a system trained on data you did not collect? Who is accountable when an algorithm misses what a human eye would have caught?

I have read those debates, participated in them, and lived them. And I can tell you from direct clinical experience: the answer is neither naive enthusiasm nor defensive rejection. The answer is exactly what Jay Patel argues across every chapter of this book, rigorous integration, structured validation, human oversight, and a values framework that places the patient at the center of every decision.

AI, in radiology as in every other specialty, is a tool. A powerful, fast, tireless, pattern-recognizing tool that can genuinely elevate the quality of clinical decision-making. But a tool requires a trained hand. A tool requires judgment about when to trust it and when to question it.

This book presents that distinction with exceptional clarity. It does not oversell AI, and it does not fear it. It demands something harder, that we build the human capability to use it wisely.

Human Verification, Human Validation: The Non-Negotiable Principle

The section of this book that I believe will have the most lasting impact, and that I would most urgently recommend to every clinical leader deploying AI systems, is its treatment of AI verification and validation.

In radiology, I read AI-generated findings every day. The systems that alert me to possible pulmonary emboli, flag potential fractures, or pre-screen mammography images for signs of malignancy are sophisticated, genuinely helpful, and sometimes extraordinary in their sensitivity. I have also seen them be confidently, clearly wrong.

This is not a failure of the technology. This is the nature of probabilistic systems operating in a world of infinite biological variation.

Jay Patel's framework for AI governance, the protocols for validation, the structured human review loops, the accountability structures, the continuous monitoring of AI performance in real clinical conditions, should be read as required learning by every hospital board, every CMO, and every physician champion responsible for clinical AI deployment.

The Crisis in Medical Education, and a Way Forward

I want to speak candidly about medical education, because this is where I believe the stakes are highest and the current systems are most urgently in need of the transformation this book describes.

The answer, which this book develops with exceptional care in its treatment of medical education reform, is both more rigorous clinical training and AI literacy that is embedded in a clinical context, not appended to a curriculum as an elective.

I was particularly moved by this book's treatment of what makes a 'world class physician.' The criteria are demanding, integrated, and right.

Humanity Is the Standard, Not the Sentiment

I want to address something that is sometimes missing in books about technology: the insistence, which pervades every chapter of this work, that humanity is not a soft counterweight to the hard logic of AI; it is the standard against which every clinical AI application must be evaluated.

In my surgical practice, I have delivered diagnoses that changed lives irreversibly. I have had the privilege of being present at moments of profound human vulnerability. I have seen what it means to a family when a clinician looks at them as people, not as cases. And I have seen the clinical consequences, in adherence, in outcome, in recovery, when patients feel seen, heard, and genuinely cared for.

Jay Patel's five pillars, AI, Technology, Quality, Leadership and Human Values, are not a hierarchy in which technology drives and values follow. Remove any one, and the structure fails. This is not philosophy. It is clinical engineering.

This book asks these questions on every page. That is what makes it different.

A Word to Those Who Will Use This Book

If you are a hospital leader, read this book as a governance framework. The chapters on AI implementation, quality management, and clinical governance give you a structured approach to one of the most consequential decisions your institution will make.

If you are a clinical educator, read this book as a curriculum challenge. The sections on medical education reform are a direct, evidence-based argument for teaching medicine differently, more practically, more humanly, more completely.

If you are a physician or surgeon, read this book as a professional development resource. The frameworks for AI verification, quality improvement, and clinical leadership will sharpen the thinking you bring to a clinical environment that is changing faster than any curriculum can track.

If you are a medical student, read this book as a description of the world you are entering, and a specification for the physician you should aspire to become. The bar this book sets is high. It should be.

And if you are a policymaker, in Delhi, in Washington, or anywhere decisions are made that shape how millions of people access healthcare, read this book as an argument for investment: in training, in quality infrastructure, in AI governance, and above all in the conviction that world-class care is not a privilege but a right.

Jay Patel has done something rare: he has written a book that is simultaneously rigorous and readable, technically detailed and genuinely human, ambitious in its vision and practical in its implementation. It reflects forty years of expertise applied with conviction to the most important challenge in healthcare today.

It deserves to be read carefully. It deserves to be acted on. And it deserves to reach every leader, educator, clinician, and student who carries any responsibility for the quality of care that patients receive. I commend it to you without reservation.

Dr. Shrenik Shah

A board-certified Vascular and Interventional Radiologist based in the Atlanta, Georgia area who specializes in minimally invasive procedures like Uterine Fibroid Embolization (UFE) and complex peripheral artery disease

Table of Contents

Preface

Building World-Class Hospitals and Medical Colleges

AI, Digital Transformation, Quality, Leadership, and Humanity

By

Dr. Bharatbhai Patel

Dean, Bhagyoday Medical College

Kadi, Gujarat, India

As Dean of Bhagyoday Medical College, I have had the privilege of shaping the minds and character of hundreds of future physicians over many years of service in medical education. In that time, I have read a great many books: textbooks, clinical references, policy frameworks, and research compendia. Very few have arrived at precisely the right moment, carrying precisely the right message, for precisely the right audience. This book is one of those rare exceptions.

The challenges facing our medical colleges today are unlike any our predecessors encountered. We are asked to produce graduates who are not only scientifically excellent, who understand pathophysiology, pharmacology, and clinical reasoning with genuine depth; but who are also humane, ethically grounded, culturally sensitive, and fully prepared to practice in an environment increasingly shaped by digital technology and artificial intelligence. That is a formidable mandate, and it demands a correspondingly formidable guide.

This book provides exactly that. In its pages, faculty members, clinical educators, and institutional leaders will find a coherent, practical, and inspiring framework for integrating the imperatives of quality, efficiency, and humanity into the educational experience of every medical student who passes through our doors.

"The measure of a great medical college is not the examinations its graduates pass, but the lives they save, the suffering they relieve, and the dignity they uphold in every patient encounter."

Quality: The Foundation That Must Not Be Negotiable

In medical education, quality is not an administrative preference; it is a moral obligation. When a student graduates without fully developed clinical competencies, the consequences are not measured in rework or customer complaints. They are measured in misdiagnoses, in delayed treatments, in patients who trusted us and were let down. This book takes that reality seriously.

The quality management frameworks presented here, rooted in globally recognized standards and adapted thoughtfully for the unique demands of medical education and healthcare delivery, offer our faculty a systematic, evidence-based methodology for ensuring that every student, in every discipline, achieves a level of competence that is fit for purpose. The integration of structured quality thinking into curriculum design, clinical training protocols, assessment methods, and institutional governance is not, as some fear, a bureaucratization of education. It is, on the contrary, the most reliable pathway to the consistent excellence our students and their future patients deserve.

I was particularly struck by the book's treatment of outcome-based quality measurement. Too often in academic medicine, we measure inputs, contact hours, library resources, faculty qualifications, and assume that outputs will follow. This book challenges that assumption with clarity and conviction, offering practical tools for measuring what actually matters: the competency, the judgment, and the professional character of the graduate.

Efficiency: Doing More for Patients, Not Less

The word 'efficiency' is sometimes met with suspicion in educational circles, as though its pursuit must come at the expense of depth, care, or humanity. This book dispels that misunderstanding beautifully. The efficiency it advocates is not the efficiency of the assembly line; it is the efficiency of the committed teacher who has structured her curriculum so carefully that not a single contact hour is wasted; of the clinical supervisor who uses case-based learning to achieve in two hours what would otherwise require a full day; of the administrator who has eliminated the bureaucratic obstacles that once prevented faculty from focusing on students.

For medical colleges operating in resource-constrained environments, as many of our institutions in Gujarat and across India must, this conception of efficiency is not a luxury but a necessity. We owe it to our students, and through them to their patients, to make the most of every resource we have. This book shows us how.

Humanity: The Irreducible Core of Medical Practice

But it is the book's treatment of humanity that I consider its most important and distinctive contribution. In an era of accelerating technological change, when artificial intelligence can read a radiograph, machine learning can flag a drug interaction, and telemedicine can connect a patient in a remote village to a specialist in Ahmedabad; it would be easy to conclude that the human dimensions of medicine are becoming less important. This book argues compellingly, and in my view correctly, that exactly the opposite is true.

The more powerful our diagnostic and therapeutic technologies become, the more the patient relies on the physician's humanity to make sense of what those technologies mean for their life, their family, and their future. The capacity for empathy, for honest communication in moments of crisis, for cultural respect, for ethical discernment under pressure, these are not soft skills at the periphery of medical competence. They are its very centre.

This book integrates the cultivation of humanity into the educational framework in a manner that is both deeply principled and practically actionable. It does not treat compassion as an innate trait that some students possess and others do not. It treats it as a professional capacity that can be modelled, practiced, assessed, and developed, in clinical simulations, in reflective practice sessions, in the structure of every student-patient encounter from the very first year of training.

"Technology can diagnose. Algorithms can analyse. Only a physician with a fully developed humanity can heal."

Patient Safety: The Ultimate Accountability

All of this, the quality, the efficiency, the humanity, converges on a single purpose: the safety and well-being of the patient. Patient safety is the lens through which every chapter of this book should be read, and it is the standard by which every graduate of every medical college must ultimately be judged.

India is building its healthcare capacity at a remarkable pace. The National Medical Commission's Competency-Based Medical Education reforms, the expansion of hospital infrastructure in semi-urban and rural areas, and the growth of telemedicine, these are transformative developments. But they can only achieve their potential if the physicians who inhabit our healthcare system have been trained to the highest standards of safety culture: to speak up when they observe a risk, to follow protocols with discipline, to communicate clearly with colleagues and patients, and to treat every near-miss as a learning opportunity rather than something to be concealed.

This book gives medical educators the tools to build that safety culture from the first days of a student's training. I commend it unreservedly for that reason.

A Word to My Fellow Faculty

To my esteemed colleagues in medical education, the professors, lecturers, demonstrators, clinical tutors, and simulation instructors who give their energy and expertise to the formation of our future doctors, I say this: read this book not as a set of mandates imposed from above, but as a conversation between peers about the work we have chosen and the standards to which we hold ourselves.

Teaching medicine is one of the most consequential acts a human being can perform. The student sitting before you today may, thirty years from now, be the physician on whom your own family depends in its most vulnerable moment. This book is an invitation to take the full weight of that reality into our classrooms, our wards, our simulation labs, and our assessment chambers, and to build, together, an educational experience equal to it.

To the students of Bhagyoday Medical College and of every institution where this book finds a home: you are entering a profession of incomparable privilege and incomparable responsibility. The knowledge, the systems, and the values in these pages are your inheritance. Honour them.

Dr. Bharatbhai Patel

Dean, Bhagyoday Medical College

Kadi, Gujarat, India

May 2026

Book Review

Authored by Jay P. Patel, ASQ Fellow I Quality & Productivity Solutions, Inc.

www.qpsinc.com

Reviewed by Dr. Bharatbhai Patel, Dean, Bhagyoday Medical College, Kadi, Gujarat

Overview

At a moment when medical education in India and globally is navigating the simultaneous demands of competency-based reform, technological disruption, and deepening expectations around patient safety and ethical practice, Jay P. Patel's book arrives as an authoritative and urgently needed guide. Written from the perspective of a practitioner with three decades of experience in quality management, operational excellence, and the integration of AI into complex organizational systems, this book bridges a gap that has long existed in the medical education literature: the gap between the world of quality science and the world of clinical teaching.

The result is a work of remarkable breadth and practical utility, one that medical college faculty, hospital administrators, curriculum designers, and institutional leaders will return to repeatedly as they navigate the transformation of their institutions in the years ahead.

Scope and Structure

The book is organized around three interlocking imperatives, quality, efficiency, and humanity, which the author correctly identifies as the defining challenges of 21st-century medical education. This framework is not merely rhetorical. It provides a coherent organizing principle that gives the work structural integrity and allows the reader to see the connections between topics that are often addressed in isolation: curriculum design, AI-enabled assessment, patient safety culture, clinical simulation, ethical formation, and institutional governance.

The opening sections establish the landscape with admirable clarity. The author situates medical education within the broader context of global quality management practice, drawing on internationally recognized frameworks, including ISO management system standards, Lean Six Sigma methodology, and competency-based outcome models, and translating them with skill and precision into language and applications that are immediately relevant to the medical college environment. This translation is itself no small achievement. Quality science and clinical education have developed largely in parallel, and the synthesis offered here is genuinely original.

The middle sections address the integration of artificial intelligence into medical education with a balance of enthusiasm and measured realism that will serve readers well. The author is neither a utopian who promises that AI will solve every challenge in healthcare and education, nor a skeptic who dismisses its potential. He is an experienced practitioner who has guided organizations through complex technological transitions, and his treatment of AI reflects that experience: grounded in what actually works, attentive to the conditions required for success, and consistently focused on how technology serves, rather than displaces, human judgment and human values.

The closing sections on patient safety, ethical formation, and the cultivation of humanity in clinical practice are, for this reviewer, the most compelling in the book. They reflect a conviction, one I share with great passion, that the purpose of all our quality systems, all our technology, and all our pedagogical innovation is ultimately the patient lying in the bed, whose life and dignity depend on the physician we have trained.

Particular Strengths

Several features of this book distinguish it from others that have addressed similar territory. First, the author writes with genuine dual fluency, in both the language of quality management and the language of medical education, which is far rarer than one might expect and which makes the work accessible to readers from both traditions. A quality professional approaching this book for the first time will find the medical education context clearly explained; a clinical educator approaching quality management will find the frameworks rendered in terms that connect directly to their daily practice.

Second, the practical orientation of the book is consistent throughout. Every conceptual framework is accompanied by tools, templates, worked examples, and implementation guidance. This is not a theoretical treatise; it is a practitioner's manual in the best sense of that term, designed to be used in the real work of building and improving a medical college or teaching hospital. Faculty facilitating workshops, department heads designing assessment systems, and deans evaluating institutional quality culture will all find material they can put to work immediately.

Third, and most importantly for this reviewer, the book never loses sight of the human being at the centre of medical practice. In a domain where quality management tools can sometimes become ends in themselves, divorced from the purposes they are meant to serve, the author consistently returns to the patient, to the student's developing character, and to the moral dimensions of clinical practice. The sections on compassion, on communication in difficult conversations, and on cultural respect and dignity in patient care are not afterthoughts appended to a systems manual. They are integral to the book's argument and to its vision of what excellent medical education achieves.

"This book does what few works in either quality management or medical education have attempted: it speaks simultaneously to the scientist who must measure and the healer who must care, and it shows convincingly that these are not competing vocations but a single calling."

Relevance for Bhagyoday Medical College and Teaching Hospitals

From the specific perspective of institutions like Bhagyoday Medical College, medical colleges in semi-urban and non-metropolitan settings serving diverse patient populations with significant primary and secondary care needs: this book is of value. The author's frameworks are explicitly designed to be scalable and adaptable, and the book addresses with sensitivity the realities of resource-constrained environments where the aspiration to world-class quality must be pursued with intelligence and discipline rather than unlimited expenditure.

The chapters addressing clinical competency development, simulation-based training, faculty development, and the measurement of educational outcomes offer teaching hospitals a rigorous and practical playbook for the continuous improvement of clinical training. The integration of patient safety culture into curriculum design is especially relevant: in settings where our graduates will be the primary, sometimes the only, physician for communities with limited access to specialist care, the safety habits and clinical judgment formed in training will directly determine patient outcomes.

I recommend this book for adoption as a core reference text for medical college faculty development programs, for use in institutional quality committees and teaching hospital governance structures, and for distribution to every clinical department head and curriculum committee member. Its systematic framework, practical tools, and unwavering ethical compass make it an ideal companion for the journey toward the highest standards of medical education and patient care.

A Note on the Author

Jay P. Patel, ASQ Fellow, is the Founder and CEO of Quality & Productivity Solutions, Inc. (QPS Inc.), a Boston-based training, consulting, and auditing firm specializing in ISO management systems, Lean Six Sigma, and the integration of artificial intelligence into quality and business processes. His credentials include the ASQ Lancaster Medal and Master Lean Six Sigma Black Belt certification, and his consulting work spans manufacturing, healthcare, regulated industries, and professional services across the United States and internationally.

What distinguishes Mr. Patel as an author in this domain is not only his technical expertise, which is substantial, but his genuine commitment to the human purposes that quality systems are designed to serve. He brings to medical education the same conviction that has guided his work across industries: that quality is not a compliance exercise but a moral commitment, and that the measure of any system is ultimately the dignity and well-being of the people it serves.

That conviction animates every chapter of this book, and it is why this reviewer regards it not merely as a useful professional resource but as a work that articulates a philosophy of educational purpose that medical colleges everywhere would do well to adopt.

Recommendation

This book is essential reading for medical college faculty, teaching hospital administrators, clinical educators, department heads, institutional quality officers, and all those charged with shaping the next generation of physicians in India and beyond. It is a rare work that is simultaneously intellectually rigorous, practically useful, and genuinely inspiring, and it arrives at a moment when the medical education community needs all three.

Dr. Bharatbhai Patel

Dean, Bhagyoday Medical College

Kadi, Gujarat, India

May 2026

Introduction

How to Use This Book

> *"Healthcare stands at a crossroads. The decisions made in the next five to ten years will shape the delivery of care for the next generation."*
>
> **From Chapter 3 the challenge that every chapter of this book addresses.**

What This Book Is

This book is a comprehensive leadership framework for the most important transformation healthcare has faced in a generation which is, the integration of artificial intelligence, digital systems, and quality management into healthcare institutions, in ways that genuinely serve patients, all patients, equitably, with excellence and with compassion.

It is practical, every chapter provides specific tools, frameworks, checklists, and real-world examples that leaders can apply directly. It is evidence-based, every recommendation is grounded in research, regulatory standards, and demonstrated practice at leading institutions in both the United States and India. And it is values-driven, because the technical and managerial dimensions of healthcare transformation are meaningless without the human values that give them purpose.

It is not a technology manual. It does not assume you are a data scientist or a software engineer. It assumes you are a leader, in a hospital, a medical college, a health system, a policy organization, or any role that shapes how healthcare is delivered, who needs to understand AI deeply enough to make wise decisions about it, and who cares enough about patients to make those decisions well.

The Structure of the Book

The book is organised into seven parts, each building on the last. You may read it from beginning to end, and this is recommended for the fullest understanding, or you may navigate directly to the parts most relevant to your immediate challenges. Each chapter opens with a clear statement of what it addresses and closes with key takeaways and a bridge to the next chapter.

PART 1 Chapters 1–3	Vision, Purpose & Humanity: The philosophical foundation, why healthcare exists, the personal journey behind this book, the global challenges that make transformation urgent, and the Mission and Core Values that govern everything that follows.
PART 2 Chapters 4–7	AI & Technology: What AI is, how it works in healthcare, its applications department by department, data as the lifeline of AI, and digital transformation, including the critical, and often neglected, topic of equipment digitization and automated data collection.
PART 3 Chapters 8–10	Quality, Excellence & Systems Thinking: The quality management framework for healthcare, patient safety, continuous improvement, Lean Six Sigma, and the integration of quality systems with AI. The chapter that demonstrates why quality governance and AI governance are the same discipline.
PART 4 Chapters 11–14	Regulations, Standards & Governance: The regulatory landscape for both the USA (HIPAA, FDA, Joint Commission, CMS) and India (NABH, NDHM/ABDM, CDSCO, Ayushman Bharat), plus global standards (WHO, ISO, HL7 FHIR), European regulations including GDPR and the EU AI Act, global medical education accreditation, and AI Ethics governance.
PART 5 Chapters 15–18 + 17A	World-Class Medical Education: Rethinking how we train physicians, the gaps in current systems, the power of AI in education, the specific criteria that define world-class doctors and world-class humans, how soft skills are taught at leading institutions globally, and faculty development for excellence.
PART 6 Chapters 19–21	Implementation, From Vision to Reality: The four-phase AI Implementation Roadmap, change management frameworks and tools,
PART 7 Chapters 22–24 + Appendices	Humanity, Leadership & the Future: Compassion in the digital age, leadership in transformation, the balanced model of AI + humanity, the global vision, and the call to action. Followed by five practical appendices: Implementation Checklist, Hospital Readiness Assessment, AI Risk Register, Quality Metrics Dashboard, and Training Programs.

How to Use This Book

Suggested Reading Pathways, Based on Your Role

- Hospital CEO / CMO / Board Member: Begin with Parts 1 and 6 (Vision and Implementation), then Part 4 (Regulations), then Part 3 (Quality). Use Parts 2 and 7 as a reference
- Quality Director / Patient Safety Leader: Begin with Part 3 (Quality & AI), then Part 2 (AI Technology), then Part 6 (Implementation). All Appendices are directly relevant
- Medical College Principal / Dean: Begin with Part 5 (Medical Education), then Part 1 (Vision and Values), then Part 4 (Regulations including NMC and NABH). Parts 6 and 7 for implementation
- Clinical Department Head / Physician Champion: Begin with Part 2 (AI Applications by department), then Part 3 (Quality), then Chapter 20 (Change Management). Appendix A (Implementation Checklist) is your working document
- Medical Student / Resident: Begin with Part 1 (Vision), then Part 5 (Medical Education and World-Class Physician Criteria), then Part 2 (AI Technology). Read the book end to end, it describes the world you are entering
- Policymaker / Health Administrator: Begin with Part 4 (Regulations USA and India), then Part 1 (Vision), then Part 6 (Implementation). Chapter 24 (The Future) is particularly relevant
- Read cover to cover, the recommended pathway: the seven parts build on each other deliberately. The reader who completes all 24 chapters will have a comprehensive, integrated understanding of healthcare AI transformation that no single-topic book can provide

A Note on the USA and India Dual Context

This book is written explicitly for both the United States and India, two countries with profoundly different healthcare systems, regulatory environments, infrastructure challenges, and patient populations, but with equally urgent needs for AI-integrated, quality-driven, human-centered transformation.

Where regulatory frameworks, accreditation standards, clinical contexts, or implementation realities differ between the two countries, this book addresses both explicitly, in side-by-side comparisons, in parallel examples, and in specific guidance for each context. Leaders in the United States will find the India-specific content valuable as a window into healthcare transformation in resource-constrained and high-volume environments. Leaders in India will find the USA-specific content valuable as a benchmark of regulatory rigour and quality management maturity.

Both will find that the underlying principles, quality management, AI governance, human values, leadership, and medical education excellence, are universal. The tools are the same. The application is adapted to the context. This is the spirit of this book: globally informed, locally adapted.

A Final Invitation

This book was written to be used: not shelved. Every framework has been designed to be applied. Every checklist is ready to be completed. Every case study is meant to prompt the question: What would this look like in my institution?

The most important response to this book is not agreement or admiration. It is action. One decision made more wisely because of something read in these pages. One AI system governed more carefully. One staff training program built with more intentionality. One medical student mentored more deliberately. One patient cared for with more genuine compassion.

Those individual actions, multiplied across the leaders who read this book and the institutions they lead, are the transformation this book is working toward.

PART ONE

Vision, Purpose & Humanity in Healthcare

Understanding why healthcare exists, and what it must always protect

Chapter 1

The Purpose of Healthcare

Why We Heal, The Foundation of Every System, Technology, and Decision

> *"The art of medicine consists of amusing the patient while nature cures the disease."*
>
> **Voltaire and yet, in the 21st century, both art and science must work together.**

1.1 Introduction: Why Purpose Matters

Before we discuss artificial intelligence, digital systems, electronic health records, or any technology, we must ask a fundamental question, one that is too often skipped in the excitement of innovation:

Why does healthcare exist?

The answer seems obvious. Yet, the way hospitals are run, the way medical schools teach, and the way technology is deployed, all reveal that this question is frequently forgotten. Systems grow large, budgets are debated, technologies are purchased, and in the middle of all this complexity, the patient, the human being at the center, can become secondary.

This chapter is a reminder. A reset. A return to the purpose that must anchor every decision in healthcare, from the policy made in a boardroom in Washington D.C. or New Delhi, to the diagnosis given in a rural clinic in Gujarat.

Healthcare is not a product. It is a promise. A promise that every human being, regardless of wealth, geography, language, or background, will receive care when they are vulnerable. Understanding and honoring that promise is the first step in any true transformation.

1.2 Healthcare as Service to Humanity

The word "hospital" is derived from the Latin word "hospitalis", meaning a place of welcome, of shelter, of refuge. For centuries, long before technology existed, healers offered what they had: knowledge, presence, and compassion. The patient came not just for a cure, but for assurance that they were not alone.

This fundamental truth has not changed.

What has changed is scale. Today, a single major hospital system in the United States may serve hundreds of thousands of patients annually. In India, government hospitals in cities like Mumbai or Delhi can see thousands of outpatients in a single day. The challenge is no longer simply healing one patient; it is building systems capable of healing millions, consistently and equitably.

Yet scale must never become an excuse for the loss of humanity. The patient who enters a hospital is not a number in a queue. They are a person carrying fear, hope, and trust. That trust, perhaps the most fragile element in all of healthcare, is both the foundation and the measure of every system we build.

The Core Promise of Healthcare

- Every patient deserves dignified, respectful, and competent care
- The healthcare system exists to serve the patient, not the other way around
- Access, equity, and compassion are not optional; they are foundational
- Technology and processes are tools to fulfill the promise, they never end in themselves
- The patient's trust is the most valuable and most fragile element in the system

1.3 Love, Compassion, and Dignity in Care

In medical schools around the world, students are trained in anatomy, physiology, pharmacology, and clinical procedures. These are essential. But how much time is spent teaching compassion? How much curriculum addresses what to say to a patient who has just received a difficult diagnosis? How to hold the hand of a family waiting outside a surgical suite? How to deliver news with honesty and kindness simultaneously?

The answer, in too many institutions, is: not enough.

Dr. Francis Peabody, a Harvard physician, wrote in 1927, nearly 100 years ago, words that remain powerfully true today: 'The secret of the care of the patient is in caring for the patient.' This is not sentimentality. It is a clinical truth. Research consistently shows that patients who feel heard, respected, and emotionally supported have better outcomes. They adhere to treatment plans. They communicate symptoms accurately. They trust their care teams.

Compassion is not a soft skill. It is a clinical tool.

In India, the concept of seva, selfless service, has for centuries defined the relationship between healer and patient. In the American healthcare tradition, the Hippocratic ideal of 'first, do no harm' carries a similar moral weight. Across cultures, the message is the same: the physician, nurse, and healthcare worker enter into a relationship of trust and responsibility that goes far beyond technical competence.

As we build AI systems and digital hospitals, we must ask: are we preserving this? Are our technologies making space for compassion, or crowding it out?

The answer depends entirely on how we design, implement, and lead these systems.

1.4 Patient-Centered Philosophy: Designing Around the Human

The phrase 'patient-centered care' has become widely used in healthcare policy and management. But what does it actually mean, in practice, every day, in the real world?

Patient-centered care means that every decision, from hospital layout to appointment scheduling, from communication protocols to treatment pathways, is designed around the patient's experience, needs, and values. Not around administrative convenience. Not around the preferences of departments. Around the patient.

In the United States, organizations like the Institute for Healthcare Improvement (IHI) and The Joint Commission have worked for decades to define and measure patient-centered care. The framework includes respect for patient preferences, coordination of care, emotional support, physical comfort, information and education, continuity, and access.

In India, the National Accreditation Board for Hospitals (NABH) has adopted similar patient-centered standards. Hospital accreditation now requires evidence not just of clinical competence, but of patient rights, informed consent, grievance mechanisms, and care coordination.

What both systems recognize is this: quality in healthcare cannot be defined without the patient's perspective.

Patient Rights	Patient Responsibilities	System Obligations
• Right to information • Right to informed consent • Right to privacy & dignity • Right to second opinion • Right to grievance redressal • Right to access records	• Provide accurate history • Follow treatment plans • Respect care team • Communicate concerns • Adhere to guidelines • Participate in decisions	• Equitable access to care • Safe environment • Skilled, compassionate staff • Clear communication • Continuous improvement • Accountability & transparency

1.5 The Role of Doctors as Healers: Not Just Professionals

In modern healthcare, the word 'professional' is used constantly. Healthcare professionals. Medical professionals. The language of professionalism emphasizes competence, standards, liability, and credentials. These are important but they are incomplete.

A professional delivers a service. A healer enters a relationship.

This distinction matters enormously, especially as AI begins to perform many tasks that were previously exclusive to trained clinicians, reading radiology images, detecting patterns in lab results, flagging medication interactions, and predicting disease risk. If doctors see themselves only as technical professionals, AI will, in many areas, outperform them. But if doctors understand themselves as healers, as human beings in a relationship of trust and responsibility with another human being, then AI becomes a tool in their hands, not a replacement for their role.

This is not anti-technology. It is pro-humanity. The future belongs to the physician who combines clinical mastery with emotional intelligence, who uses AI to enhance their capabilities while never allowing it to replace their judgment, their empathy, or their presence.

In both the United States and India, the medical profession is under pressure. Physician burnout is at record levels. In the U.S., studies show that more than 50% of physicians report symptoms of burnout. In India, doctors in public health systems often carry patient loads that are simply unsustainable. This pressure erodes the very humanity we are trying to protect.

Sustainable healthcare, both systems and individuals, requires that we address these structural realities. AI can help. Efficient processes can help. But ultimately, healthcare systems must invest in the wellbeing of their healers as seriously as they invest in their equipment.

What Makes a Great Healer, Universal Qualities

- Clinical expertise: Deep, current, evidence-based knowledge
- Compassion: The ability to understand and share another's suffering
- Integrity: Honesty with patients, families, and colleagues, always
- Humility: Knowing the limits of one's knowledge and seeking help
- Communication: The ability to translate complexity into understanding
- Resilience: Sustaining excellence under pressure, day after day
- Curiosity: A commitment to lifelong learning and improvement

1.6 Real-World Reflection: Two Healthcare Worlds

Consider two patients on a single day: one in Chicago, Illinois, and one in Ahmedabad, Gujarat.

In Chicago, a 58-year-old woman with chest pain is brought to a Level 1 trauma center. She is triaged within minutes. An ECG is read by an AI-assisted algorithm while a cardiologist reviews simultaneously. A stent is placed within 90 minutes of arrival. The hospital's electronic health record has her complete history. The care coordinator will arrange follow-up before she leaves.

In Ahmedabad, a 62-year-old farmer presents to a government hospital with similar symptoms. He has waited since 5 AM. There are three doctors for 400 patients today. His records, a folder of handwritten notes he carries in a plastic bag, are incomplete. The cardiologist, if available, may see him in hours. There is no AI, no integrated record system, no care coordinator.

Both patients are human beings with equal dignity and equal need. The gap between their experiences is not inevitable. It is a gap in systems, resources, training, and political will. It is a gap that technology, properly implemented, can help close. But only if we first agree that both patients deserve the same quality of care, the same dignity, the same promise.

This book is written for leaders who are committed to closing that gap, in the United States, in India, and everywhere in between.

1.6 Our Mission: World-Class Healthcare for Every Person

> *"World-class is not a destination. It is a daily decision, made by leaders, teachers, clinicians, and every person who touches a patient's life."*
>
> **Jay P. Patel, Quality & Productivity Solutions, Inc.**

The mission that drives this book is simple to state, and demanding to live:

To build and sustain world-class healthcare systems, through the disciplined training of people, the transformation of culture, and the continuous application of innovation, quality tools, and improvement techniques, so that every patient, everywhere, receives the best care possible.

This is not a corporate mission statement written for a wall. It is a working commitment, one that has been tested across thirty years of quality management consulting, across industries and continents, and is now being applied, with full conviction, to the most human of all sectors.

Three forces make this mission urgent right now. First, the technology exists, AI, digital systems, predictive analytics, that can fundamentally elevate healthcare quality at scale. Second, the knowledge exists: Lean, Six Sigma, systems thinking, evidence-based management, that can make improvement systematic and sustainable. Third, and most critically, the need exists: billions of people in the United States, India, and across the world still do not receive the quality of care they deserve.

The gap between what is possible and what is delivered is not a gap in technology. It is a gap in trained people, educated communities, and transformed cultures. Closing that gap is the mission.

Mission Statement

To advance world-class healthcare in the United States and India

by training and educating healthcare leaders, clinicians, and communities;

by transforming organizational culture through discipline, values, and accountability;

and by applying the best innovation, quality tools, and improvement techniques

so that every patient receives safe, compassionate, and excellent care

every time, everywhere, for everyone.

1.7 Core Values: The Non-Negotiables

Core values are not aspirations. They are not marketing language. They are the non-negotiable standards of behavior, decision-making, and leadership that define who we are, as individuals, as institutions, and as a healthcare community. Every policy, every training program, every AI system, and every patient interaction in this book is governed by these five values.

1	**COMPASSION, We care deeply about every person.** Every patient, student, staff member, and community member we serve is a human being deserving of respect, dignity, and empathy. Compassion is not background noise in our work; it is the foreground. It is the reason every tool, technique, and training program in this book exists. We teach it. We measure it. We model it. In a world increasingly mediated by screens and algorithms, we protect the human heart of healthcare.
2	**EXCELLENCE, World-class is the only standard we accept.** Adequate is not acceptable. Good enough is not good enough. Whether we are training a nurse in Ahmedabad, implementing an AI diagnostic tool in Chicago, or designing a medical school curriculum in Gujarat, we apply the same global benchmark: world-class. This means evidence-based practices, measurable outcomes, structured processes, and the relentless pursuit of better, not as a project, but as a permanent operating philosophy. Excellence requires training, reinforcement, accountability, and leadership that models the standard it expects from others.
3	**INTEGRITY, We do what is right, even when it is difficult.** Integrity in healthcare means telling patients the truth. It means reporting errors so systems can improve. It means implementing AI with transparency, so patients and clinicians understand how decisions are being supported. It means leaders who model accountability rather than deflecting blame. In a field where lives depend on trust, integrity is not optional. It is the foundation on which every relationship, between patient and provider, between institution and community, is built.
4	**INNOVATION, We embrace better ways, always.** Innovation is not about technology alone; it is about the courage and discipline to continuously question how things are done and seek better answers. Lean tools, Six Sigma methods, AI systems,

	simulation-based training, digital health platforms, these are all expressions of the same commitment: to never accept the status quo when improvement is possible. In healthcare, innovation saves lives. We embed a culture of innovation through structured training, protected time for improvement projects, leadership support for new ideas, and the systematic sharing of what works across teams and institutions.
5	**EQUITY, World-class care belongs to everyone.** A farmer in rural Gujarat and an executive in suburban Chicago share the same fundamental right: access to safe, quality healthcare. Equity means designing systems that close gaps, in access, in outcomes, in opportunity, rather than systems that simply serve those who are already advantaged. AI, when implemented with equity as a design principle, can extend world-class capability to underserved communities. Training programs must reach frontline workers, not just senior leaders. Education must reach the community, not just the classroom. Equity is not charity. It is justice, and it is the true measure of a world-class system.

1.8 Guiding Principles: How the Values Become Action

Core values answer the question: what do we believe? Guiding principles answer the question: how do we behave? These principles translate the five values above into specific, observable commitments that govern every aspect of healthcare training, education, system design, and leadership described in this book.

Guiding Principle 1, Training Is Not Optional: It Is the Engine of World-Class Care
• Every healthcare worker, from the surgeon to the housekeeper, must be trained to the highest standard that their role demands. Training is not a one-time event. It is a continuous, structured system: onboarding, ongoing skill development, cross-training, and leadership development • In both USA and India, under-trained staff is the single most preventable cause of quality failures and patient harm • Training programs must include technical skills, quality tools, AI literacy, communication, ethics, and patient-centered care • Investment in training is an investment in patient safety; it is the highest-return expenditure a healthcare institution can make
Guiding Principle 2, Education Transforms Communities, Not Just Individuals
• World-class healthcare cannot exist in a community that does not understand health, prevention, and how to navigate the system • Medical education must prepare future doctors who are technically brilliant, humanly compassionate, and systemically aware • Community health education, in schools, workplaces, and rural settings, reduces disease burden and emergency care demand • Faculty development is as important as student education: trained, passionate, innovative teachers produce great doctors • The medical college and the hospital are not separate institutions; they are one ecosystem of learning and healing
Guiding Principle 3, Culture Change Is the Hardest and Most Important Work

- Technology can be purchased in a month. Culture takes years to change, and must be led, not mandated
- A culture of quality means every team member owns outcomes, reports problems, and continuously seeks improvement
- Culture change requires visible leadership commitment, consistent modeling of values, and genuine accountability for behavior
- Fear-based cultures suppress reporting and learning, the exact opposite of what patient safety requires
- A culture that celebrates improvement, that sees a reported near-miss as a learning opportunity, not a failure, is the highest form of organizational excellence

Guiding Principle 4, Innovation and Improvement Are Structured Disciplines, Not Random Events

- Lean, Six Sigma, PDCA, A3 problem-solving, FMEA, root cause analysis, these are not acronyms. They are life-saving tools
- AI is a powerful new tool in this tradition; it must be implemented with the same rigor as any quality improvement initiative
- Improvement must be measured: what cannot be measured cannot be managed, and what cannot be managed cannot be improved
- Every department, every team, every role must have improvement targets, structured review processes, and authority to act
- Sharing what works, across departments, institutions, and countries, multiplies the impact of every improvement made

TRAIN	EDUCATE	TRANSFORM
Every person, every role	*Students, faculty & community*	*Culture, systems & outcomes*
Clinical skills	Future doctors	Quality culture
Quality tools	Faculty development	Safety systems
AI literacy	Community health	AI integration
Communication	Health literacy	Continuous improvement
Leadership	Lifelong learning	World-class outcomes

This is the operating model of transformation. Not technology alone. Not a single training event. Not a memo from leadership. But a sustained, structured, values-driven cycle: Train the people, Educate the community, Transform the culture, deliver world-class care, Measure outcomes, Improve again. Every chapter of this book contributes to one or more of these three pillars.

★ KEY TAKEAWAYS

1. Healthcare's purpose is to serve human life with dignity, compassion, and competence. This must anchor every decision. Transformation requires more than planning, it requires the courage to build
2. Patient-centered philosophy means designing every system, process, and technology around the patient's needs and values.
3. Compassion is not a soft skill; it is clinically proven to improve outcomes and must be formally taught and sustained.
4. Doctors are healers first, professionals second. AI augments human care but cannot replace human relationships.
5. Our Mission: world-class healthcare through training people, educating communities, and transforming culture, everywhere, for everyone.
6. Five Core Values, Compassion, Excellence, Integrity, Innovation, and Equity, are non-negotiable and govern every decision in this book.
7. Four Guiding Principles drive action: Training is the engine, Education transforms communities, Culture change is the hardest work, Innovation is a structured discipline.
8. The operating model: Train people, Educate community, Transform culture, Deliver world-class care, Measure, Improve. Always.

▶ COMING NEXT

Chapter 2 tells the personal story behind this book, how one journey from a small village in India to global consulting shaped a philosophy of healthcare transformation. Understanding where these ideas come from helps explain why they matter so deeply.

Chapter 2

My Journey: From Village to Global Vision

How One Life's Path Became a Framework for Healthcare Transformation

> *"Education is the most powerful weapon which you can use to change the world."*
>
> **Nelson Mandela, a truth lived, not just quoted, in the villages of Gujarat.**

2.1 Introduction: Why Personal Stories Matter in Leadership

Every philosophy has an origin. Every framework has a foundation. And every leader who drives meaningful change in complex systems does so, consciously or not, from a deeply personal place.

The values formed in scarcity: discipline, humility, the belief that learning can change a life, are precisely the values that failing healthcare systems need most. And the systems thinking learned across decades of consulting, in factories, in corporations, in quality management, is exactly what healthcare institutions need to build the kind of AI-integrated, patient-centered systems this book envisions.

Great ideas do not emerge from abstract theory alone. They emerge from lived experience, applied carefully to real challenges.

2.2 Thol: Where the Journey Began

Thol is a small village near Ahmedabad in the state of Gujarat, India. It is perhaps best-known today for the Thol Lake Bird Sanctuary, a quiet, beautiful wetland that attracts migratory birds and, increasingly, tourists. But for the families who lived and farmed there in the mid-twentieth century. It was a place of simple, difficult living. My parents were farmers. They tilled the land, grew crops, and raised their family with the tools available to them: hard work, honesty, deep moral values, and the conviction that their children could have a better life if they were educated. They did not have university degrees. They had something more durable: clarity of purpose and strength of character.

The resources we had were few. But the lessons I absorbed in that environment were profound:

- Work completely. Whatever you do, give it your full effort, not because someone is watching, but because excellence is its own standard.
- Live honestly. Integrity is not situational. It does not change when conditions are difficult.
- Respect every person. The farmer, the teacher, the shopkeeper, every human being carries dignity.
- Education is the path. Not just schooling, but the relentless pursuit of knowledge that transforms what is possible.

These are not just the lessons of a childhood in rural India. They are the principles that underlie every quality management system, every leadership framework, and every healthcare transformation this book will describe.

2.3 The Power of Education and Discipline

Education, in the environment in which I grew up, was not taken for granted. It was pursued with intention and sacrifice. Long study hours were not a burden; they were an investment. This discipline of learning, not just absorbing information, but applying it, questioning it, and building on it, became the foundation of everything that followed.

From village schooling, the path led to engineering education in India, and then, through ambition and hard work, to advanced studies in the United States, a Master's degree and an MBA. Each step required adapting to new environments, new expectations, and new ways of thinking. Each step required what every healthcare system today also requires: the willingness to learn, change, and improve.

The MBA opened doors to understanding organizations, how they succeed, how they fail, what leadership actually requires in practice. The engineering foundation provided something equally important: a systems mindset. The belief that problems are not random, that root causes can be found, that processes can be improved, and that excellence can be made systematic rather than accidental.

Lessons from a Learning Journey, Applied to Healthcare

- Discipline creates consistency: The same discipline that builds a student's knowledge builds a hospital's quality culture
- Systems thinking reveals root causes: Engineering habits of mind are exactly what healthcare improvement requires
- Adaptability is a strength: The ability to learn in new environments is the core competency of transformation leaders
- Investment in learning pays compound interest: Educated, trained staff consistently outperform untrained ones, in every sector
- Humility enables growth: The best learners, and the best leaders, know how much they do not yet know

2.4 Thirty Years of Quality Work: What Industry Teaches Healthcare

After completing education in the United States, a career in quality management, productivity improvement, and organizational consulting began, one that has now spanned more than three decades and taken me to organizations across industries and continents.

Working with manufacturing companies, technology firms, service organizations, and government institutions, I have observed one truth repeated in every sector, every culture, and every size of organization:

The principles of quality are universal. What makes a factory excellent, clear processes, trained people, measured outcomes, continuous improvement, leadership commitment, is exactly what makes a hospital excellent. The tools have different names. The terminology differs. But the underlying logic is identical.

Lean manufacturing teaches waste elimination. In a hospital, wasted steps mean delayed care. Six Sigma teaches variance reduction. In a hospital, uncontrolled variance means inconsistent patient outcomes. Root Cause Analysis teaches us not to blame individuals but to fix systems. In hospitals, blame culture kills improvement before it starts.

Over thirty years, I have seen factories transform, going from chronic defects and delays to world-class performance, through the disciplined application of these principles. I have seen organizations grow, cultures change, and people exceed their own expectations of what was possible.

Healthcare can do the same. It must do the same.

2.5 Expanding the Mission: Why Healthcare, Why Now

The decision to focus significantly on healthcare was not made in a conference room. It came from experience, from walking through hospitals in Gujarat and USA, consulting with medical institutions, and observing, with both admiration and concern, what I saw.

I saw dedicated doctors working 14-hour days with a genuine commitment to their patients. I saw nurses navigating outdated systems with extraordinary professionalism. I saw administrators trying to manage complex organizations with limited tools and data. And I saw patients, real human beings, experiencing a system that was, in many ways, working against its own best intentions.

At the same time, I was observing the global rise of artificial intelligence. Not as a distant technology, but as a present reality already transforming radiology, genomics, drug discovery, and operational management in leading hospitals worldwide. The convergence was clear: healthcare needed what quality management and AI together could provide. And healthcare leadership needed guidance that connected technology to strategy, and strategy to human values.

The vision for Bhagyoday Hospital and Medical College in Kadi, Gujarat, is to build a fully digital, AI-enabled, patient-centered healthcare and education ecosystem.

2.6 What This Journey Teaches Every Healthcare Leader

Healthcare leaders today, whether in the United States or India, whether running a 20-bed community hospital or a 2,000-bed tertiary care center, are facing a moment of historic transformation. The decisions they make in the next five to ten years will shape healthcare for the next generation.

These decisions will require technical knowledge, understanding AI, data systems, and regulatory frameworks. But more than technical knowledge, they will require what every great leader in every field has always required: clarity of purpose, strength of character, commitment to continuous learning, and the humility to keep asking whether what they are building truly serves the people it is meant to serve.

Village Lessons	Career Lessons	Healthcare Lessons
• Work with full effort • Live with integrity • Respect all people • Education transforms • Values are durable • Purpose drives action	• Systems reveal root causes • Quality is measurable • Culture enables change • Leadership drives results • Data informs decisions • Improvement never ends	• Patient trust is fragile • Technology serves people • Compassion is clinical • Training is non-negotiable • AI amplifies human skill • Vision requires courage

2.7 Real-World Reflection: The Bhagyoday Vision

Bhagyoday, in Gujarati, the word carries the meaning of rising fortune, of a new dawn. It is a fitting name for a project that represents exactly what this book is about: the convergence of vision, technology, quality, and human values in service of a community.

The vision for Bhagyoday Hospital and Medical College is not simply to build a modern facility. It is to demonstrate that world-class, AI-integrated, patient-centered healthcare can be achieved in a semi-urban Indian context, and that the model can then be replicated and scaled across regions.

This means: paperless operations, AI-assisted diagnostics, fully integrated EMR systems, Lean-managed processes, NABH-accredited quality standards, AI literacy for every staff member and student, and an ethical governance framework that ensures technology serves patients rather than displacing human care.

It is an ambitious vision. It is also a necessary one. Because the world does not need more incremental improvement in healthcare. It needs transformation. And transformation requires leaders willing to build, not just plan.

★ KEY TAKEAWAYS

9. Personal values formed early, discipline, integrity, respect, and the love of learning, are the foundation of effective leadership.
10. Thirty years of quality management across industries confirms: the principles that make factories excellent make hospitals excellent.
11. Healthcare needs leaders who combine technical knowledge with human wisdom, and AI with genuine compassion.
12. The Bhagyoday vision demonstrates that world-class AI-integrated healthcare is achievable in developing contexts, if leadership commits.
13. Every healthcare leader must ask: What is the personal foundation from which I lead? Are my values aligned with the purpose of healthcare?
14. Transformation requires more than planning; it requires the courage to build, to experiment, to learn, and to keep going.

▶ COMING NEXT

Chapter 3 looks forward to the global challenges healthcare faces, the emerging role of technology, and the vision of what world-class healthcare systems can become. The journey from village to global vision now points toward the future.

It was a place of simple, hard life.

Chapter 3

The Future of Healthcare

Global Challenges, Technological Possibilities, and the Vision of World-Class Care

> *"The greatest danger in times of turbulence is not the turbulence; it is to act with yesterday's logic."*
>
> **Peter Drucker, a management visionary whose wisdom applies to every healthcare system today.**

3.1 Introduction: Standing at a Crossroads

Healthcare systems around the world are at a crossroads. On one side lies the familiar: the old models, the paper-based processes, the fragmented systems, the hierarchy-driven culture that has characterized healthcare for generations. On the other side lies a future that is arriving faster than most institutions are ready for: AI-driven diagnostics, genomic medicine, predictive analytics, digital therapeutics, robotic surgery, and patient empowerment through real-time data.

The question is not whether this future is coming. It is coming. The question is who will shape it, and whether it will be shaped in ways that serve all of humanity, or only the privileged few.

This chapter maps the global challenges that make transformation urgent, explores the possibilities that technology is opening, and presents a vision of what world-class healthcare systems, in the United States, in India, and globally, can and must become.

3.2 Global Challenges in Healthcare

To understand why transformation is necessary, we must first honestly confront the scale of the challenges facing healthcare worldwide. These are not small problems. They are systemic, interconnected, and urgent.

Challenge 1: Access and Equity

The most fundamental challenge in global healthcare is that it is not global. Access to quality care remains profoundly unequal, between nations, within nations, between urban and rural populations, and between economic classes.

In the United States, despite being the world's largest economy, approximately 25 million people remain uninsured, and millions more are underinsured. Life expectancy varies by more than 20 years depending on zip code. Racial and ethnic disparities in healthcare outcomes, in maternal mortality, in cardiovascular disease, in cancer survival, are persistent and well-documented.

In India, where 1.4 billion people rely on a healthcare system that is still developing its infrastructure, the challenges are different in nature but equally profound. The doctor-to-patient ratio in rural India is severely inadequate. Specialist care is concentrated in major urban centers. Out-of-pocket healthcare expenses are the leading cause of catastrophic poverty for millions of Indian families each year.

Challenge 2: Rising Burden of Non-Communicable Disease

Globally, non-communicable diseases (NCDs), cardiovascular disease, diabetes, cancer, and chronic respiratory conditions, account for approximately 74% of all deaths worldwide, according to the World Health Organization. These are largely preventable and manageable conditions. Yet they continue to overwhelm healthcare systems because those systems are built for acute care, not chronic disease management.

India now has more than 77 million people living with diabetes, the second highest in the world after China. The United States faces its own NCD epidemic, with obesity, hypertension, and diabetes driving enormous healthcare costs and human suffering. Managing these conditions requires a shift from episodic, reactive care to continuous, proactive, data-driven care. AI makes this shift possible. But it requires both the technology and the systems to deploy it effectively.

Challenge 3: Workforce Stress and Burnout

Healthcare workers around the world are under extraordinary pressure. The COVID-19 pandemic dramatically worsened a problem that was already serious: physician and nurse burnout at epidemic levels, staff shortages, moral injury from working in systems that cannot meet demand, and high rates of mental health challenges among frontline workers.

This is not simply a human resources challenge. It is a patient safety challenge. Fatigued, burned-out clinicians make more errors. High staff turnover destroys institutional knowledge and care continuity. And a healthcare system that does not take care of its people cannot, ultimately, take good care of its patients.

Challenge 4: Data Fragmentation and Poor Information Systems

Despite decades of effort and billions of dollars of investment, most healthcare systems still struggle with basic data management. Patient records are fragmented across multiple providers and systems. Information does not follow the patient. Critical data is unavailable at the point of care. Clinical decisions are made without the full picture.

In the United States, despite widespread adoption of Electronic Health Records (EHRs), interoperability, the ability of different systems to share data seamlessly, remains a serious challenge. In India, the National Digital Health Mission (NDHM) is working to create a unified health ID system, but implementation at scale is still in progress. Until data flows freely and securely between providers, the promise of AI in healthcare cannot be fully realized.

The Four Global Healthcare Crises Requiring Urgent Action
• Access and equity: 4.5 billion people globally lack access to essential health services (WHO, 2023) • Rising NCDs: 74% of global deaths from preventable non-communicable diseases • Workforce crisis: 40+ million healthcare worker shortage projected globally by 2030 • Data fragmentation: Most healthcare systems still cannot share patient data across providers

3.3 Technology as a Response: What Is Now Possible

The good news, and it is genuinely good news, is that the same era that has produced these challenges has also produced the tools to address them. Artificial intelligence, when properly implemented within quality-driven systems and guided by ethical leadership, offers transformative possibilities for healthcare.

AI-Powered Diagnostics

AI algorithms trained on millions of medical images can now detect diabetic retinopathy, breast cancer on mammograms, pulmonary nodules on CT scans, and skin lesions with accuracy that matches or exceeds trained specialists in controlled studies. In contexts where specialist access is limited, rural India, underserved communities in the US, AI-powered diagnostic tools can democratize access to expert-level interpretation.

FDA-cleared AI diagnostic tools are already deployed in hospitals across the United States. In India, initiatives like the National AI for Health program are beginning to bring similar capabilities to government health facilities. The technology is ready. The implementation challenge, training, trust, governance, infrastructure, is where leadership makes the difference.

Predictive Analytics and Early Warning Systems

AI systems trained on patient vital signs, laboratory values, medication records, and clinical notes can predict, with significant accuracy, which patients are likely to deteriorate in the next hours, which patients are at high risk of sepsis, and which patients are likely to be readmitted within 30 days. These predictive capabilities allow clinical teams to intervene before crises occur, rather than responding after they do.

This shift, from reactive to predictive care, is one of the most important transformations that AI enables. It is also one of the most concrete ways in which AI can reduce both patient harm and healthcare costs simultaneously.

Operational AI: Efficiency at Scale

Beyond clinical applications, AI is transforming hospital operations. Intelligent scheduling systems reduce wait times and optimize resource utilization. AI-powered supply chain management reduces waste and ensures that critical supplies are available when needed. Automated administrative processes, billing, coding, documentation, reduce the burden on clinical staff and decrease administrative errors.

In both the United States and India, administrative costs represent a significant proportion of total healthcare expenditure. AI-driven automation can reduce these costs substantially, freeing resources for direct patient care.

3.4 Technology vs Human Connection: The Essential Balance

And yet, and this is perhaps the most important point in this chapter, technology alone does not create better healthcare.

Every experienced clinician knows that some of the most important moments in healthcare happen in the space between the data and the patient. The moment when a doctor sits down, closes the laptop, and says: 'Tell me what is worrying you most.' The moment when a nurse notices that something is not right about a patient, not from the monitors, but from years of experience and observation. The moment when a family receives difficult news, and the physician's presence, truly present, not distracted, makes an unbearable situation somehow more bearable.

No AI system, no matter how sophisticated, can replace these moments. They are irreducibly human. And they are clinically important. The risk in the enthusiasm for digital transformation is not that we will adopt too much technology; it is that we will fail to protect the spaces where human connection does its essential work.

The world-class healthcare system of the future will not be one in which doctors are replaced by algorithms. It will be one in which doctors are freed from repetitive, low-value tasks, documentation, retrieving data, and routine monitoring, so that they can do more of what only humans can do: think holistically, decide under uncertainty, communicate with compassion, and be present for their patients.

This is the balanced model that this book advocates. Not technology versus humanity, but technology serving humanity.

3.5 Vision: What World-Class Healthcare Systems Look Like

Let us be specific about what we are building toward. The world-class healthcare system of the future, whether in Houston, Texas, or Kadi, Gujarat, shares the following defining characteristics:

Fully Digital and Interconnected

Every patient has a secure, portable, longitudinal health record. Information flows freely and securely between providers, across specialties, and across institutions. AI has access to complete, high-quality data. Patients have access to their own records and can share them easily with any provider they choose.

Predictive and Preventive

The system identifies risk before disease manifests. Population health analytics flag individuals at high risk of developing chronic conditions. Preventive interventions are deployed proactively. Emergency departments manage predictable volumes because chronic disease is being managed in the community, not in crises.

Equitable and Accessible

Geography is not destiny. Technology extends specialist expertise to rural and underserved areas through telemedicine and AI-powered tools. Financial barriers are minimized through intelligent insurance systems and government programs. Language and literacy barriers are addressed through AI translation and simplified communication.

Quality-Driven and Safe

Every clinical process is standardized to evidence-based best practice. Variation is monitored and managed. Near-misses are reported and analyzed. Continuous improvement is embedded in culture, not imposed from the outside. Safety is everyone's responsibility, and systems are designed to make the safe choice the easy choice.

Human-Centered and Compassionate

Despite all technology, the patient remains at the center. Staff are trained not just in clinical skills but in communication, empathy, and patient engagement. Burnout is actively managed. Culture supports both clinical excellence and human flourishing, for patients and providers alike.

Globally Informed and Locally Adapted

The best practices from healthcare systems around the world, the coordination models of Denmark, the quality systems of Singapore, the cost management of Thailand, the preventive programs of Cuba, the innovation ecosystems of the United States, are studied, adapted, and implemented in the local context. No system has all the answers. Every system has something to teach.

Vision Framework: The World-Class Healthcare System

- Digital infrastructure: Unified EHR, real-time data access, secure interoperability
- AI integration: Diagnostic AI, predictive analytics, operational automation
- Quality systems: Evidence-based protocols, continuous improvement, safety culture
- Regulatory compliance: HIPAA/FDA (USA), NABH/NDHM (India), ISO global standards
- Workforce development: AI literacy, compassion training, burnout prevention
- Patient empowerment: Access to records, shared decision-making, health literacy
- Ethical governance: AI ethics committee, bias monitoring, accountability frameworks
- Financial sustainability: Cost-efficient models accessible to all socioeconomic levels

3.6 Real-World Reflection: The Road to Bhagyoday

The vision described in this chapter is not abstract. It should be built, step by step, decision by decision,

The journey began with a simple question: What would it look like to build healthcare in this community the right way, not just adequately, but excellently? Not just for the patients who can afford it, but for everyone? Not just using today's tools, but designed for the future?

The answer required confronting both the global best practices described in this chapter and the specific realities of semi-urban Gujarat: the patient population's needs, the available workforce, the infrastructure, the regulatory environment, and the cultural context.

What emerged is a phased implementation plan that begins with foundational digital infrastructure, moves through AI integration and quality system development, and ultimately aims for full NABH accreditation and a model that can be studied and replicated across the region.

It is a long journey, but it is the right journey. And it begins, as all meaningful journeys do, with a clear vision of where you are going and an honest assessment of where you are now.

The chapters that follow will give you the knowledge, frameworks, and tools to build your own version of this vision, wherever you lead, regardless of the scale or context. The principles are universal. The application is yours to make.

★ KEY TAKEAWAYS

15. Healthcare stands at a crossroads, between legacy systems that are failing and technological possibilities that are transformative.
16. Four urgent global crises demand action: inequitable access, rising NCDs, workforce burnout, and data fragmentation.
17. AI offers genuine solutions, in diagnostics, predictive analytics, and operational efficiency, but only when properly implemented.
18. The essential balance is technology serving humanity, not replacing the human moments that define great care.
19. World-class healthcare systems share six defining characteristics: digital, predictive, equitable, quality-driven, compassionate, and globally informed.
20. This vision is achievable in real contexts, not just aspirational, but practical and buildable.
21. The leader's role is to hold both the vision and the reality simultaneously, and to close the distance between them, systematically and courageously.

▶ COMING NEXT

Part 2 of this book turns to the technology itself. Chapter 4 begins with a clear, accessible explanation of Artificial Intelligence, what it is, how it works, the different types of AI relevant to healthcare, and how it compares to human intelligence. Understanding the technology is the foundation for using it well.

PART TWO

AI & Technology in Healthcare

Understanding the tools, the data, and the digital infrastructure that will transform care

Chapter 4

Understanding Artificial Intelligence

What It Is, How It Works, and Why Healthcare Leaders Must Know It

> *"Artificial intelligence is not a substitute for human intelligence; it is a tool to amplify human capability."*
>
> **Fei-Fei Li, AI pioneer at Stanford University**

4.1 Introduction: Why Every Healthcare Leader Must Understand AI

You do not need to be a data scientist to lead an AI transformation in healthcare. But you do need to understand what AI is, what it can do, what it cannot do, and how it makes decisions. A leader who cannot answer these questions cannot evaluate AI vendors intelligently, cannot protect patients from algorithmic harm, and cannot build the trust that AI adoption requires among clinicians and staff.

This chapter is written for leaders, not programmers. Every concept will be explained in plain language, with healthcare examples. By the end of this chapter, you will be able to hold a substantive conversation with your technology team, ask the right questions of AI vendors, and begin building the AI literacy that your entire organization needs.

That last point is critical: AI literacy is not just for leaders. It is for every person in your healthcare organization from the radiologist interpreting AI-assisted scans, to the nurse using a predictive risk tool, to the administrator managing an AI-optimized scheduling system.

One of the four Guiding Principles established in Chapter 1 is that innovation and improvement are structured disciplines. Building AI literacy throughout your organization is where that principle begins.

4.2 What Is Artificial Intelligence? A Simple Definition

Artificial Intelligence (AI) refers to the capability of computer systems to perform tasks that normally require human intelligence, such as recognizing patterns, making decisions, understanding language, and learning from experience.

The keyword in that definition is learning. Traditional computer programs follow explicit rules written by programmers: if this happens, do that. By contrast, AI systems can learn patterns and rules from data They improve their performance over time as they are exposed to more examples. This ability to learn from data, rather than following only pre-programmed rules, is what makes AI fundamentally different from earlier software, and what makes it so powerful in complex domains like healthcare.

AI in Plain Language: Three Everyday Comparisons
• Email spam filter: learns from millions of examples of spam vs. legitimate email to correctly classify new messages, without being explicitly programmed with spam rules • Netflix recommendations: learns your viewing patterns and those of similar users to predict what you will enjoy, improving with every show you watch • AI in radiology: learns from millions of labeled X-rays, MRIs, and CT scans to detect abnormalities, improving as more cases are reviewed and validated by radiologists

4.3 Types of AI Relevant to Healthcare

AI is not one technology; it is a family of related approaches, each suited to different kinds of problems. Healthcare leaders need to understand three main categories: Machine Learning, Deep Learning, and Generative AI.

Machine Learning (ML)

Machine Learning is the broadest category of AI. It encompasses algorithms that learn patterns from labeled data and use those patterns to make predictions or decisions on new, unseen data. ML is the engine behind most practical AI applications in healthcare today.

In healthcare, ML is used to predict patient readmission risk, identify patients likely to develop sepsis, flag medication interactions, optimize appointment scheduling, and detect billing fraud. These applications share a common structure: the system is trained on historical data (thousands or millions of past patient records), learns which patterns are associated with which outcomes, and then applies that learning to new patients in real time.

The critical requirement for ML to work is data quality. Garbage in, garbage out, this old computing principle has never been truer than in AI. If the training data is incomplete, biased, or inaccurate, the ML model's predictions will also be biased or inaccurate. This is why Chapter 6 of this book, on data as the lifeline of AI, is one of the most important chapters for healthcare leaders to internalize.

Deep Learning (DL)

Deep Learning is a specialized subset of Machine Learning that uses artificial neural networks, computational systems loosely inspired by the structure of the human brain, to analyze data with extraordinary depth and complexity. Deep Learning excels at tasks involving images, audio, and other high-dimensional data that simpler ML algorithms struggle to process.

In healthcare, Deep Learning is the technology behind AI systems that can read medical images. A Deep Learning model trained on hundreds of thousands of chest X-rays can detect pneumonia, tuberculosis, and lung nodules with accuracy that rivals, and in some specific tasks, exceeds, trained radiologists. The same technology is being applied to pathology slides (detecting cancer cells), retinal photographs (screening for diabetic retinopathy), and ECG recordings (identifying arrhythmias).

Deep Learning requires enormous amounts of training data and significant computing power. This is why the best medical AI systems have been built by large institutions and technology companies with access to massive datasets. For smaller hospitals, the practical path is to adopt validated, FDA-cleared or CDSCO-approved Deep Learning tools developed by others, rather than attempting to build from scratch.

Generative AI

Generative AI represents the newest and most rapidly developing frontier of AI. Rather than simply classifying or predicting based on existing patterns, Generative AI creates new content, text, images, code and audio, that did not previously exist. The most prominent examples are large language models (LLMs) like Claude, GPT-4, and Google Gemini, which can generate fluent, contextually accurate text on virtually any topic.

In healthcare, Generative AI is already being applied to automate clinical documentation (converting physician voice notes into structured clinical records), generate patient-friendly discharge summaries, assist in medical education through interactive case simulations, support drug discovery by generating and evaluating molecular structures, and provide first-level triage support through intelligent patient-facing chatbots.

Generative AI also carries unique risks that healthcare leaders must understand: it can generate plausible-sounding but factually incorrect information (a phenomenon called hallucination), it can reflect biases present in its training data, and its outputs require human review before clinical use. These risks are manageable, but only by leaders and clinicians who understand them.

Machine Learning	Deep Learning	Generative AI
• Learns from labeled historical data • Predicts outcomes & risk scores • Sepsis prediction, readmission risk • Medication interaction flagging • Fraud detection, scheduling optimization • Requires quality data & validation • Most widely deployed in healthcare today	• Neural networks for complex data • Excels at images, audio, and signals • Radiology image analysis • Pathology slide interpretation • ECG & EEG pattern detection • Requires large datasets & computing power • Best adopted via validated commercial tools	• Creates new content from patterns • Large language models (LLMs) • Clinical documentation automation • Patient education materials • Medical education simulations • Risk: hallucination, requires oversight • Fastest-growing AI category

4.4 AI vs Human Intelligence: Understanding the Difference

One of the most important, and most misunderstood, aspects of AI is how it differs from human intelligence. This understanding is essential for healthcare leaders because it determines where AI should be trusted, where it should be used with caution, and where human judgment must always prevail.

What AI Does Well	What Human Intelligence Does Better
Processes enormous volumes of data rapidly and consistently	Integrates context, emotion, and relationship into clinical judgment
Detects subtle statistical patterns invisible to the human eye	Applies moral reasoning and ethical judgment to complex situations
Performs the same task at the same quality level at 3 AM as at 9 AM	Navigates ambiguity, uncertainty, and novel situations without training data
Monitors hundreds of patients simultaneously without fatigue	Communicates with compassion, reads body language, builds trust
Applies evidence-based guidelines consistently across all patients	Knows when to break the protocol because this patient is different
Learns from millions of cases across many hospitals simultaneously	Draws on lived experience, intuition, and mentorship
Never forgets a guideline, never misreads a drug name due to tiredness	Recognizes the human being behind the diagnosis

The critical insight from this comparison is not that AI is better or worse than human intelligence; it is that they are different in nature and complementary in practice. The physician who uses AI to catch what they might miss and uses their human intelligence to do what AI cannot is more capable than either alone. The healthcare system that understands this and designs its AI implementation accordingly will achieve results that neither pure human practice nor AI alone could produce.

4.5 AI as Decision Support: The Critical Principle

The most important principle governing the use of AI in clinical settings is one that must never be compromised: AI supports decisions. It does not make them.

In every clinical AI application, from a sepsis prediction alert to an AI-assisted radiology read to a medication recommendation, the final decision authority rests with the trained, licensed, accountable human clinician. This is not merely a legal or regulatory requirement (though it is both). It is the correct way to use AI in a domain where errors have life-or-death consequences and where individual patient circumstances can always diverge from statistical patterns.

What does this mean in practice? It means that AI outputs must always be presented to clinicians as information to consider, not instructions to follow. It means that clinicians must be trained to interrogate AI recommendations, to ask why the system flagged a particular patient, what data it used, and whether that recommendation makes sense given everything they know about this specific patient. It means that over-reliance on AI, sometimes called automation bias, must be actively counteracted through training and culture.

The Decision Support Hierarchy: Who Decides What

- AI system: detects patterns in data, generates recommendations, flags risks, and presents options
- Clinical team: reviews AI output in the context of the full patient picture: history, values, preferences, clinical examination
- Senior clinician / attending physician: makes the final clinical decision with full accountability
- Patient: participates in shared decision-making, informed by the clinical team's synthesis of all information including AI input
- This hierarchy is non-negotiable, AI is never the final decision-maker in clinical care

4.6 Technology and Systems: The AI Ecosystem in Healthcare

AI in healthcare does not operate in isolation. It functions within a broader technology ecosystem that must be understood by healthcare leaders. The components of this ecosystem, and how well they work together, determine whether AI delivers its promised benefits or falls short.

Electronic Health Records (EHR/EMR): The Data Foundation

AI cannot function without data. The Electronic Health Record (EHR) or Electronic Medical Record (EMR) is the primary source of patient data on which most clinical AI systems are trained and within which they operate. A hospital without a robust, comprehensive, well-maintained EHR system is not ready for AI, regardless of what any vendor claims.

In the United States, EHR adoption accelerated dramatically after the HITECH Act of 2009 incentivized adoption. Today, the major EHR platforms, Epic, Cerner, Meditech, Allscripts, are deeply embedded in American hospital operations. The challenge has shifted from adoption to optimization: ensuring that EHR data is structured, complete, and accessible to AI tools.

In India, EHR adoption is more uneven. Leading private hospital groups: Apollo, Fortis, Max Healthcare, have implemented sophisticated EHR systems. Government hospitals and smaller private facilities often still operate on paper or basic digital systems. The National Digital Health Mission (NDHM) aims to create a unified health ID and digital health infrastructure for all Indians, but full implementation will take years. Healthcare leaders in India must build their digital foundation now, not wait for the national system to mature.

Clinical Decision Support Systems (CDSS)

Clinical Decision Support Systems are software tools that provide clinicians with patient-specific information, filtered and presented at appropriate times, to enhance patient care. AI-powered CDSS represents the most direct application of AI at the point of care, embedded within clinical workflows so that recommendations appear when and where clinicians need them.

Examples include: drug-drug interaction alerts that fire when a potentially dangerous combination is ordered, sepsis prediction scores that appear in the nurse's view when a patient's vital signs begin trending toward deterioration, imaging AI that highlights areas of concern on a radiology read, and antibiotic stewardship tools that recommend de-escalation when culture results are available.

The key design challenge for CDSS is alert fatigue, when systems generate so many alerts that clinicians begin dismissing them without reading. World-class CDSS implementation requires careful calibration: high-sensitivity alerts for the most critical situations, suppression of low-value alerts, and continuous monitoring of alert response rates to ensure the system is being used as intended.

Interoperability: Making Systems Talk to Each Other

An AI system is only as good as the data it receives. When patient data is fragmented across multiple non-communicating systems: different EHRs at different hospitals, separate lab systems, disconnected pharmacy records, paper-based specialty notes, AI tools are operating with incomplete information. Their recommendations may be missing critical context.

The healthcare industry has developed technical standards to address this: HL7 (Health Level Seven) defines messaging standards for exchanging health information, and FHIR (Fast Healthcare Interoperability Resources) provides a modern, web-based framework for data sharing. In the United States, the 21st Century Cures Act requires EHR vendors to support FHIR-based data sharing. In India, the NDHM has adopted FHIR as its data exchange standard.

For hospital leaders, interoperability means asking a non-negotiable question of every technology vendor: Does your system support HL7 FHIR? And ensuring that your own EHR infrastructure is configured to share and receive data through these standards. Interoperability is not a technical nicety; it is the prerequisite for AI to work safely and effectively.

4.7 AI Literacy: Building It Across Your Organization

A critically important but frequently neglected aspect of AI implementation is organization-wide AI literacy. The most sophisticated AI system will fail if the people who use it, manage it, or are affected by it do not understand what it is and how it works.

AI literacy does not mean everyone becomes a data scientist. It means:

- Frontline clinicians understand what AI can and cannot do, and how to critically evaluate AI recommendations
- Nurses and allied health professionals know how to interpret AI-generated risk scores and when to escalate
- Administrators understand AI's role in operations and can evaluate performance metrics meaningfully
- Leaders can make informed decisions about AI procurement, governance, and ethics
- Patients are informed about how AI is used in their care and can ask meaningful questions

Building this literacy requires structured training programs, not a single orientation session, but ongoing education woven into professional development. It requires champions at every level who model AI-critical thinking. And it requires a culture that encourages questions about AI recommendations rather than blind deference.

This is not a one-time investment. As AI evolves, and it is evolving faster than any technology in healthcare history, AI literacy programs must evolve with it. The organization that builds AI literacy today will build its competitive and quality advantage for the decade ahead.

★ KEY TAKEAWAYS

1. AI is the ability of computer systems to learn from data and perform tasks normally requiring human intelligence; it is a tool, not a replacement for human judgment.
2. Three types matter most in healthcare: Machine Learning (predictions and risk), Deep Learning (image analysis), and Generative AI documentation, medical education, and drug discovery
3. AI and human intelligence are complementary, not competitive, AI excels at pattern detection and scale; humans excel at judgment, compassion, and context.
4. The non-negotiable principle: AI supports decisions, it never makes them. Final clinical authority always rests with the licensed human clinician.
5. The AI ecosystem requires a strong EHR foundation, Clinical Decision Support Systems, and interoperability via HL7 FHIR standards.
6. AI literacy must be built across every level of the organization, from medical students to frontline nurses to board members, through structured, ongoing training.
7. Training before deployment, not after: no AI system delivers value in the hands of people who do not understand it.

▶ COMING NEXT

Chapter 5 moves from understanding AI to applying it department-by-department across the hospital. You will see how AI is transforming radiology, the ICU, outpatient services, and hospital administration, and how to envision an integrated AI-enabled hospital model.

Chapter 5

AI & Technology Applications in Healthcare

Department- by- Department, From Radiology to Administration to the Integrated AI Hospital

> *"The best way to predict the future is to invent it."*
>
> **Alan Kay, computer scientist. In healthcare, AI is not a prediction; it is an invention already in progress.**

5.1 Introduction

AI in healthcare is not a future possibility. It is a present reality, already deployed in leading hospitals across the United States and, increasingly, across India. Radiology departments are using AI to detect cancer earlier. ICUs are using AI to predict deterioration before it becomes critical. Emergency departments are using AI to prioritize triage. Pharmacies are using AI to catch dangerous drug combinations. And hospital administrators are using AI to manage everything from staffing levels to supply chain inventory.

This chapter takes you department by department through the most important AI applications in healthcare today. For each area, you will find: what the AI does, what the evidence shows, what implementation requires, and how the application fits into a world-class, patient-centered system. The chapter closes with a vision of the fully integrated AI hospital, not as a futuristic concept, but as a practical goal for forward-thinking institutions in both the United States and India.

5.2 Radiology: The AI Success Story

Radiology is the most mature and evidence-rich domain for AI in healthcare. The reason is structural: radiology generates vast quantities of standardized, digital image data, exactly the kind of data that Deep Learning algorithms excel at analyzing. The results have been remarkable.

AI systems have now demonstrated accuracy equal to or exceeding that of trained radiologists in specific tasks: detecting diabetic retinopathy in retinal photographs (Google Health), identifying breast cancer in mammograms (DeepMind/NHS), detecting pulmonary nodules in CT scans, classifying skin lesions, and identifying intracranial hemorrhage in CT brain scans. These are not laboratory results; they are validated in real clinical settings with real patient data.

What AI Does in Radiology

- Automated detection: flags areas of concern on X-rays, CT scans, MRIs, and ultrasound images for radiologist review
- Prioritization: ensures that urgent findings (hemorrhage, pneumothorax, large vessel occlusion) are surfaced to the top of the radiologist's worklist, reducing critical result turnaround time
- Quantification: measures tumor size, tracks changes between scans, calculates bone density: tasks that are time-consuming for humans and prone to measurement variation
- Report generation: AI assists in drafting preliminary radiology reports, which radiologists then review, edit, and sign, reducing documentation burden
- Population screening: in low-resource settings, AI enables screening programs where specialist radiologist access is limited

USA and India Context

In the United States, FDA-cleared AI tools from companies like Aidoc, Viz.ai, Nuance, and Subtle Medical are deployed in hundreds of hospitals. Reimbursement codes for AI-assisted imaging interpretation are evolving, and major radiology professional societies have issued guidance on AI implementation.

In India, where the radiologist-to-population ratio is approximately 1 per 100,000 people (compared to 1 per 8,000 in the US), AI-powered radiology has transformative potential. Companies like Qure.ai (Mumbai) have developed AI tools specifically validated on Indian patient populations, designed for deployment on standard clinical infrastructure. Government programs are piloting AI-assisted chest X-ray interpretation for tuberculosis screening, a disease that kills more than 400,000 Indians annually.

Radiology AI, Implementation Checklist for Hospital Leaders

- Ensure your PACS (Picture Archiving and Communication System) is digital and integration-ready
- Evaluate AI tools that are FDA-cleared (USA) or CDSCO-approved (India) and validated on populations similar to yours
- Involve radiologists in vendor selection, clinical acceptance requires clinical ownership
- Pilot with one modality (e.g., chest X-ray) before expanding to the full department
- Define performance metrics: sensitivity, specificity, turnaround time, radiologist and override rate
- Train all radiologists and technicians on the AI tool, not just on how to use it, but on how to critically evaluate its outputs
- Monitor for bias: ensure the AI performs consistently across patient demographics in your population

5.3 The ICU: AI for the Critically Ill

The Intensive Care Unit is one of the most data-rich and highest-stakes environments in medicine. A single ICU patient may generate thousands of data points per hour: continuous vital signs, ventilator settings, laboratory values, medication infusion rates, and nursing assessments. No human clinician, regardless of skill and experience, can simultaneously always process all of this data for all patients.

This is where AI provides some of its most powerful and best-validated benefits in clinical care.

Sepsis Prediction

Sepsis, a life-threatening response to infection, kills approximately 11 million people globally each year. Early recognition and treatment are critical: for every hour of delay in appropriate antibiotic administration, mortality increases by approximately 7%. AI-powered sepsis prediction systems, like the Epic Sepsis Model and commercial tools from companies like Dascena, analyze continuous streams of vital signs, laboratory values, and clinical data to predict sepsis 6-12 hours before clinical recognition, giving care teams a critical head start.

Implementation requires integration with the EHR, clear protocols for how nurses and physicians respond to sepsis alerts, and careful threshold calibration to balance sensitivity (catching real cases) against specificity (avoiding alert fatigue from false positives).

ICU Early Warning Systems

Beyond sepsis, AI-powered early warning systems in the ICU can predict cardiac arrest, respiratory failure, acute kidney injury, and ventilator-associated complications hours before clinical deterioration becomes obvious. These systems work by learning the subtle patterns that precede deterioration from thousands of past cases, patterns too complex and multivariable for human recognition in real time.

In both US and Indian ICUs, the practical benefit is twofold: earlier intervention saves lives, and nurses can be alerted to which patients need immediate attention rather than spending equal time on all patients regardless of risk trajectory.

AI in Mechanical Ventilation

AI systems are now being applied to optimize mechanical ventilation, one of the most complex and consequential interventions in critical care. Algorithms can recommend ventilator settings based on continuous analysis of patient respiratory mechanics, adjust weaning protocols based on predicted readiness for extubation, and alert clinicians when current settings are likely to cause ventilator-induced lung injury. In India, where ICU intensivist staffing is limited, AI-assisted ventilator management has particular potential to improve outcomes.

5.4 Outpatient Department (OPD): AI at the Front Door

The Outpatient Department is where most patients first enter the healthcare system, and where AI has enormous potential to improve efficiency, accuracy, and patient experience, particularly in the high-volume OPD environments common in Indian public hospitals.

AI-Powered Triage

In emergency and outpatient settings, AI-assisted triage tools use structured patient-reported symptoms, vital signs, and demographics to recommend triage priority levels. This supports nurses and triage staff, particularly in high-volume environments, to identify which patients need immediate attention and which can safely wait. In Indian government hospitals where a single triage nurse may face hundreds of patients daily, AI assistance can be transformative for both safety and throughput.

AI in Primary Care and Chronic Disease Management

AI tools are being developed and deployed to support primary care physicians in managing chronic diseases, diabetes, hypertension, asthma, COPD, that represent many outpatient encounters. These tools analyze patient data between visits, identify patients whose disease control is deteriorating, recommend medication adjustments based on evidence-based protocols, and generate patient-specific education materials.

In both the US and India, AI-supported chronic disease management programs have demonstrated improved glycemic control in diabetic patients, better blood pressure management in hypertensive patients, and reduced emergency department visits and hospitalizations, the most expensive and disruptive form of care for patients with manageable chronic conditions.

Intelligent Appointment Scheduling and Queue Management

In high-volume OPD environments, particularly in India, where a single specialist may see 100-150 patients in a day, intelligent AI scheduling systems can dramatically improve both efficiency and patient experience. These systems learn appointment duration patterns by doctor, specialty, and visit type; predict no-show probability and adjust scheduling; accordingly, manage dynamic queue reordering based on patient acuity; and send automated reminders that have been shown to reduce no-show rates by 20-40%.

5.5 Hospital Administration: The Invisible AI

Much of the most impactful AI in healthcare operates not in the clinical domain, where it is visible to patients and clinicians, but in the administrative and operational domain, where it quietly optimizes the systems that support care delivery.

Workforce & Staffing	Supply Chain & Finance	Quality & Safety
• Predictive census modeling, forecasts patient volume by unit and shift • AI-optimized nursing staff scheduling, matches staffing to predicted demand • Turnover risk prediction, identifies staff at risk of leaving, enabling proactive retention	• Automated inventory management, predicts supply needs and prevents stockouts • Pharmaceutical demand forecasting, reduces waste from expired medications • AI-assisted medical coding, reduces billing errors and claim rejections • Revenue cycle optimization,	• Real-time patient safety monitoring, flags care gaps across all patients • Infection surveillance, detects healthcare-associated infection clusters • Readmission prediction, identifies high-risk patients for discharge planning

• Credential & competency tracking, ensures all staff certifications are current • Overtime reduction through better shift optimization	identifies claim denials and appeals opportunities • Contract analysis for vendor negotiations	• Complaint and feedback analysis, AI reads patient satisfaction data to identify patterns • Accreditation documentation support

5.6 The Integrated AI Hospital: A Vision and a Roadmap

The department-specific applications described in this chapter represent the current state of AI deployment in healthcare. But the most powerful vision, and the direction that world-class healthcare systems are moving toward, is the integrated AI hospital: an institution where AI is not a collection of separate departmental tools, but a unified, organization-wide intelligence layer that enhances care at every point.

What Integration Means

In an integrated AI hospital, data flows seamlessly across departments, the AI system managing ICU early warning has access to the same patient record as the AI tool supporting the OPD physician and the AI algorithm reviewing the radiology image. Recommendations from different AI systems are synthesized and presented coherently to clinical teams. Administrative AI and clinical AI work from the same data foundation. And the institution continuously learns: every clinical outcome, every near-miss, every variation in practice feeds back into the AI model improvement.

The Bhagyoday Integrated Model

The vision for Bhagyoday Hospital is precisely this integrated model. The system is designed so that from the moment a patient registers, whether in person or digitally, their data begins flowing through an integrated intelligence layer. Their risk profile is continuously updated. Their care team receives proactive alerts. Their discharge planning begins on admission. Their follow-up is automated and intelligent. The administrative systems managing staffing, supplies, and finance are connected to the same data environment as the clinical systems.

This is not a fantasy; it is an architecture. And it is built on the foundation of three things: a comprehensive, high-quality EHR; robust data governance; and organization-wide AI literacy. All three are addressed in the chapters that follow.

Integrated AI Hospital, The Seven Defining Characteristics

- Unified data: one patient record, accessible across all departments and AI systems in real time
- Predictive care: proactive identification of risk before deterioration, at every stage of the patient journey
- Intelligent workflows: AI optimizes the flow of patients, staff, and supplies across the institution continuously
- Closed-loop learning: clinical outcomes feed back into the AI model improvement automatically
- Human-centered design: AI is invisible to patients and supportive (never intrusive) to clinicians
- Ethical governance: an AI ethics committee oversees every AI system with defined accountability
- Continuous measurement: AI performance is monitored in real time, with clear escalation paths for underperformance

★ KEY TAKEAWAYS

1. AI in healthcare is not a future promise; it is a present reality already transforming radiology, ICU care, outpatient services, and hospital administration.
2. Radiology is the most mature AI domain: validated tools for imaging analysis are FDA/CDSCO-cleared and deployable now, especially impactful in India, where specialist access is limited.
3. ICU AI for sepsis prediction and early warning systems saves lives by detecting deterioration 6-12 hours before clinical recognition, every hospital should evaluate these tools.
4. OPD AI in triage, chronic disease management, and scheduling improves both patient outcomes and operational efficiency in high-volume settings.
5. Administrative AI in staffing, supply chain, and revenue cycle optimization is often the fastest path to measurable ROI from AI investment.
6. The integrated AI hospital, unified data, predictive care, closed-loop learning, ethical governance, is the goal: build toward it department by department.
7. Involve clinical staff in AI selection and implementation from the beginning, clinical ownership determines clinical adoption.

▶ COMING NEXT

Chapter 6 addresses the foundation that makes all of this possible: data. Without high-quality, well-governed data, no AI system can perform reliably. This chapter shows healthcare leaders how to build and manage the data infrastructure that AI requires.

Chapter 6

Data: The Lifeline of AI

How to Collect, Govern, and Trust the Information That Powers Healthcare Intelligence

> *"In God we trust. All others must bring data."*
>
> **W. Edwards Deming, the father of quality management, whose principles apply now more than ever to AI in healthcare.**

6.1 Introduction: Why Data Is the Most Critical Asset in AI Healthcare

Before a hospital deploys its first AI system, before it selects a vendor, before it trains its staff; it must ask a hard and honest question: Is our data ready?

This question is asked too rarely. Healthcare organizations across the United States and India invest in sophisticated AI tools and then discover, often expensively, that the tools cannot deliver their promised results because the underlying data is incomplete, inconsistent, biased, or inaccessible. The AI vendor is not at fault. The data is.

W. Edwards Deming, whose quality management philosophy is the foundation of this book's approach, taught that improvement requires data, and that decisions made without data are decisions made on opinion. In healthcare AI, this principle is absolute. The algorithm is only as intelligent as the data on which it is trained and the data it receives in real time. Understanding, building, and governing high-quality healthcare data is not a technical task delegated to the IT department. It is a leadership responsibility.

6.2 The Healthcare Data Landscape

Healthcare generates more data than almost any other industry, and historically, that data has been among the least effectively used. Understanding what data exists, where it comes from, and why it is so complex to work with is the starting point for building the data infrastructure that AI requires.

Structured Data

Structured data is information stored in defined fields and formats that computers can easily read, search, and analyze. In healthcare, structured data includes: demographic information (age, gender, diagnosis codes), laboratory results (numerical values with reference ranges), vital signs (recorded as numbers), medication orders (drug name, dose, route, frequency), and billing codes (ICD-10, CPT codes).

Structured data is the foundation of most clinical AI today. Machine learning models are trained on structured data extracted from EHR databases. Sepsis prediction models, readmission risk scores, and early warning systems all run primarily on structured data. The quality of this data, its completeness, accuracy, and timeliness, directly determines AI model performance.

Unstructured Data

Unstructured data is information that does not fit into predefined database fields, and it constitutes approximately 80% of all healthcare data. Clinical notes, physician dictations, nursing assessments, operative reports, discharge summaries, patient-reported symptom descriptions, radiology reports, and pathology interpretations are all unstructured. This data is extraordinarily rich in clinical meaning; but it requires Natural Language Processing (NLP)-based AI to extract that meaning in a form that other AI systems can use.

Generative AI and advanced NLP are making unstructured clinical data increasingly accessible for AI analysis. This is one of the most active areas of healthcare AI development, and one of the most important, because the insights locked in clinical notes often contain the nuance and context that structured data fields cannot capture.

Imaging Data

Medical images, X-rays, CT scans, MRIs, ultrasounds, pathology slides, retinal photographs, dermatology photographs, represent a massive and rapidly growing category of healthcare data. A single CT scan can generate hundreds or thousands of individual images. A large hospital may perform thousands of imaging studies per day. This data is the training ground for Deep Learning AI in radiology and pathology.

Imaging data requires specialized storage infrastructure (PACS, Picture Archiving and Communication Systems), standardized formats (DICOM, Digital Imaging and Communications in Medicine), and significant computing resources for AI analysis. For hospitals in India where PACS adoption is still growing, building the imaging data infrastructure is often a prerequisite for imaging AI.

Wearable and Remote Monitoring Data

A rapidly growing category of healthcare data comes from outside the hospital: wearable devices, remote patient monitoring systems, patient-reported outcomes collected via mobile apps, and continuous glucose monitors. This data provides a continuous window into patient health between clinical encounters, exactly the kind of data needed for proactive, preventive AI-driven care.

In the United States, CMS reimbursement for remote patient monitoring has expanded significantly, driving adoption. In India, affordable wearable devices are reaching populations that have never had consistent health monitoring. Integrating this data into the EHR and making it accessible to AI systems is a near-term challenge and a long-term opportunity.

6.3 Data Quality: The Make-or-Break Factor

The most important concept in healthcare AI data management is data quality. An AI model trained on poor-quality data will generate poor-quality predictions, and in healthcare, poor predictions have consequences measured in patient outcomes, not just business metrics.

Data quality in healthcare has five dimensions, each of which must be actively managed:

1	COMPLETENESS: Is all required data present? Missing values, a common problem in healthcare data, force AI models to make assumptions or exclude patients from analysis. Incomplete medication lists, missing vital signs, and absent laboratory values all degrade model performance.
2	ACCURACY: Is the data correct? Data entry errors, miscoded diagnoses, transposed laboratory values, and incorrect medication doses all create noise that degrades AI model training. Data validation rules, dual-entry verification for critical values, and regular data audits are essential.
3	CONSISTENCY: Is the same information represented the same way across systems and time? When blood pressure is recorded differently in different nursing stations, or when diagnosis codes are applied inconsistently by different physicians, AI models learn inconsistency rather than clinical truth.
4	TIMELINESS: Is data available when the AI system needs it? A sepsis prediction model that receives laboratory results 4 hours after they are obtained, because of manual data entry delays, cannot provide the early warning it was designed to give. Real-time AI requires real-time data.
5	REPRESENTATIVENESS: Does the training data reflect the population the AI will serve? An AI model trained primarily on data from urban teaching hospitals may perform poorly when deployed in rural community hospitals. A model trained on US patient populations may not transfer accurately to Indian patient populations without validation and retraining.

6.4 EMR/EHR Systems: Building the Data Foundation

The Electronic Medical Record (EMR) or Electronic Health Record (EHR) is the central repository of patient data: and therefore, the central foundation of healthcare AI. For hospital leaders, understanding what a world-class EHR implementation looks like is essential for AI readiness.

EHR Readiness for AI, USA Context	EHR Readiness for AI, India Context
Major platforms: Epic, Cerner, Meditech, Allscripts, most have built-in AI capabilities or AI app marketplaces	Platforms: Practo, Insta HMS, eVitalRx, government ABDM-compliant systems, varying AI integration maturity
21st Century Cures Act mandates FHIR-based interoperability, enforced by ONC	NDHM (National Digital Health Mission) driving standardization, adoption at early-to-mid stage
Challenge: EHR optimization, data is digital but not always clean, complete, or AI-ready	Challenge: EHR adoption, many hospitals still paper-based or using basic digital systems
AI opportunity: leverage rich existing EHR data for advanced analytics and clinical decision support	AI opportunity: build AI-ready EHR infrastructure from the start, leapfrog legacy system problems
Key requirement: API access for AI vendor integration and continuous data pipelines	Key requirement: standardized data entry protocols, staff training, and data governance framework

6.5 Data Governance: The Leadership Framework

Data governance is the framework of policies, processes, roles, and standards that ensures healthcare data is managed as a strategic asset, with defined accountability for quality, security, privacy, and appropriate use. In the context of AI, data governance is not optional: it is the mechanism by which leaders ensure that AI systems are fed accurate, representative, ethically sourced data, and that the outputs of those systems are trustworthy.

The Seven Pillars of Healthcare Data Governance

- Data ownership: defined accountability for each category of data, who is responsible for its accuracy and completeness
- Data standards: organization-wide agreement on how data is collected, coded, and formatted, the foundation of consistency
- Data quality management: regular audits, validation rules, and improvement cycles for data accuracy and completeness
- Data security: protection of patient data against unauthorized access, technical controls, access management, audit trails
- Privacy compliance: adherence to HIPAA (USA), PDPB/IT Act (India), and applicable international standards for patient data rights
- Data access and sharing: clear policies for who can access what data, under what conditions, and through what technical mechanisms
- AI model governance: oversight of how data is used to train AI models, including bias auditing, performance monitoring, and retraining protocols

Data governance requires a designated leader, often a Chief Data Officer (CDO) or Chief Information Officer (CIO), and a cross-functional data governance committee that includes clinical, technical, legal, and administrative representation. It requires written policies, defined processes, and regular review. And it requires a culture in which data quality is everyone's responsibility, from the physician who completes their clinical note accurately and on time, to the nurse who enters vital signs with precision, to the coder who assigns diagnosis codes correctly.

6.6 Data Ethics: The Principles That Protect Patients

Data in healthcare is not neutral. It is deeply personal, often sensitive, and potentially consequential. The patient who shares their health information with a healthcare provider is extending a profound act of trust, a trust that healthcare institutions have an absolute obligation to honor.

Three ethical principles govern healthcare data management in the AI era:

- Patient consent and transparency: patients have the right to know how their data is being used, including whether it is being used to train AI models. Informed consent frameworks must be updated for the AI era, and patients must have meaningful options to opt out of non-clinical data uses.
- Data minimization: AI systems should use only the data that is necessary for their intended purpose. Collecting data beyond what is needed creates unnecessary privacy risk and erodes patient trust without clinical benefit.
- Algorithmic fairness: AI systems must be regularly audited for bias, in their training data, in their outputs, and in their real-world impact across patient demographic groups. An AI system that performs well for the majority populations but poorly for minority, rural, or low-income patients is not an acceptable implementation of world-class healthcare values.

★ KEY TAKEAWAYS

8. Data is the lifeline of AI, no AI system can perform reliably on poor-quality data. Data readiness must be assessed before any AI deployment.
9. Healthcare data exists in three main forms: structured (EHR fields), unstructured (clinical notes), and imaging, each requiring different management and AI approaches.
10. The five dimensions of data quality: completeness, accuracy, consistency, timeliness, and representativeness, must all be actively managed.
11. EHR systems are the central data foundation. Both USA and India face different but equally urgent EHR readiness challenges that leaders must address.
12. Data governance is a leadership responsibility, not an IT task. It requires defined ownership, standards, security, privacy compliance, and AI model oversight.
13. Data ethics principles, patient consent, data minimization, and algorithmic fairness, are non-negotiable in the AI era.
14. Build the data foundation before deploying AI, this sequencing is the difference between AI that delivers value and AI that disappoints.

▶ COMING NEXT

Chapter 7 addresses the broader digital transformation of which data and AI are both part: how to build a fully digital hospital, paperless, cloud-enabled, interoperable, and secure. This is the infrastructure layer that makes the AI hospital possible.

Chapter 7

Digital Transformation in Hospitals

From Paper to Paperless, Building the Infrastructure of World-Class, AI-Ready Healthcare

> *"It is not the strongest of the species that survives, nor the most intelligent; it is the one most adaptable to change."*
>
> **Charles Darwin whose insight, applied to healthcare institutions, is the defining leadership challenge of our era.**

7.1 Introduction: Digital Transformation Is Not About Technology

The single most common mistake healthcare leaders make when embarking on digital transformation is believing it is primarily a technology project. It is not. Digital transformation is a people project, a culture project, and a leadership project, that happens to require technology.

Technology can be purchased. A new hospital information system can be installed in months. Cloud infrastructure can be configured in weeks. But changing the way 2,000 people work, the habits, the workflows, the assumptions, the resistances, the fears, takes years of sustained, skilled, values-driven leadership.

This chapter gives you both dimensions: the technology you need to understand and the leadership approach required to make it work. Both are essential. A hospital that invests only in technology will have an expensive digital failure. A hospital that builds culture without the right technology will have committed, motivated staff using inadequate tools. World-class digital transformation requires both, in the right sequence, with the right leadership, and always in service of the ultimate goal: better patient care.

7.2 Equipment Digitization & Automated Data Collection: The Prerequisite Nobody Talks About

There is a conversation that is almost never had in healthcare digital transformation planning, and its absence is responsible for more failed implementations than any other single factor. That conversation is this: before a hospital can go paperless, before it can deploy AI, before it can build any meaningful intelligence layer, every piece of clinical equipment that generates patient data must be computerized, networked, and configured to transmit that data automatically and in real time.

A paperless hospital is not achieved by giving staff tablets and scanning old paper records. It is achieved when the vital signs monitor sends readings directly to the EHR without a nurse re-entering them. When the ventilator streams its settings and waveforms automatically. When the laboratory analyzer reports results electronically within minutes of completion. When the infusion pump logs every medication delivery without manual documentation. When every diagnostic device speaks a digital language that the hospital's information systems understand.

This is not a technology nicety. It is the physical foundation of the entire digital transformation. Without it, staff will spend their time manually transcribing from analog or disconnected devices into digital systems, which defeats the purpose of digitization, introduces transcription errors, creates time delays that undermine clinical decision support, and makes AI-powered care impossible.

The Equipment Digitization Imperative: What Every Department Needs

Equipment digitization must be assessed and planned department by department. The following categories represent the minimum digital capability required across a world-class hospital, whether in Houston, Texas, or Kadi, Gujarat.

Department / Equipment	Minimum Digital Requirement	Data Generated & Auto-Transmitted
ICU / Critical Care	Networked patient monitors with HL7 output; ventilators with digital data ports; smart infusion pumps with EHR integration; continuous pulse oximetry with auto-logging	Vital signs every 1–5 min, ventilator settings & alarms, drug infusion rates & totals, SpO2 trends, all to EHR in real time
Emergency Department	Digital triage workstations; networked vital sign monitors; electronic medication dispensing units (Pyxis/Omnicell); ECG machines with digital transmission	Triage scores, vitals, medication dispensing records, 12-lead ECG auto-filed to EHR within 60 seconds of acquisition
Radiology & Imaging	Full PACS (Picture Archiving & Communication System); DICOM-compliant modalities, X-ray, CT, MRI, ultrasound; RIS (Radiology Information System) integrated with EHR	All images auto-uploaded to PACS in DICOM format; radiology orders auto-generated from EHR; results auto-filed when reported
Laboratory (Pathology)	Networked laboratory analyzers (chemistry, hematology, microbiology, coagulation); LIS (Laboratory Information System) with bidirectional EHR interface	All results transmitted electronically within minutes of analysis completion; critical values auto-alert to ordering clinician
General Wards / Nursing	Bedside vital sign monitors with HL7 integration; barcode medication administration (BCMA) scanners; electronic nursing documentation terminals	Scheduled vitals auto-charted; every medication administration barcode-verified and electronically recorded with timestamp and nurse ID
Operating Theatre	Anesthesia workstations with electronic record export; surgical sponge counting systems;	Complete anesthesia record auto-generated; intraoperative vitals,

	intraoperative monitoring with auto-logging	medications, and events logged in real time to HER
Pharmacy	Automated dispensing cabinets; barcode verification systems; electronic prescribing integration; robotic dispensing where feasible	Every dispense electronically recorded; medication reconciliation automated; controlled substance tracking complete and auditable
Outpatient / Clinic	Digital sphygmomanometers, glucometers, spirometers, and weighing scales with data transmission; point-of-care testing devices with LIS integration	Clinic vitals and POC results auto-populated into visit record; no manual transcription from device to system

What 'Automated' Really Means: The No-Manual-Transcription Rule

The word 'automated' in automated data collection has a precise meaning that must be enforced as a non-negotiable standard. It means: from the moment a clinical measurement is taken by a device, to the moment it appears in the patient's EHR, no human being manually re-enters or transcribes that data. Not a nurse. Not a technician. Not a clerk.

This sounds obvious. In practice, it is violated constantly, and each violation is a patient safety risk and a data quality problem. When a nurse reads a blood pressure from an analog device and types it into a computer, that number can be transposed, misread, or entered in the wrong patient's record. When a lab technician manually enters an analyzer result into the LIS, errors occur. When a radiology technician re-types patient demographics into a DICOM worklist, mismatches happen. These are not hypothetical risks; they are documented causes of patient harm.

The No-Manual-Transcription Rule, Implementation Standards

- Every device that measures a clinical parameter must have a digital output port or wireless transmission capability, no analog-only devices in a digital hospital
- Every device must be registered in the hospital's device management system with a unique identifier that links its data to the correct patient automatically
- Bidirectional interfaces are preferred: the EHR sends patient demographics and orders to the device; the device sends results back, eliminating manual patient identification at both ends
- All automated data transmissions must include: timestamp (to the second), device ID, operator ID, patient identifier, and result/value with units
- Exception handling must be defined: what happens when a device fails to transmit? Manual entry is the fallback, but must be flagged, audited, and minimized
- Regular interface testing and monitoring: automated data flows must be tested weekly and monitored continuously for failures or delays

The Hospital Equipment Readiness Assessment

Before beginning any digital transformation, every hospital leader should conduct a structured Equipment Readiness Assessment. This is a department-by-department audit of current equipment, its digital capability, its connectivity status, and the gap between where it is and where it needs to be for paperless operations.

Assessment Question	Ready	Partial	Not Ready	Action Required
Does every clinical device have digital output capability?	All devices digital	Most digital, some analog	Majority analog	*Replace/upgrade analog devices, budget and prioritize by patient impact*
Are all devices networked (wired or Wi-Fi)?	All connected	Most connected	Minimal networking	*Install hospital-grade Wi-Fi infrastructure; network all devices by department*
Do device interfaces transmit to EHR automatically?	Full auto-transmission	Partial integration	All manual entry	*Engage EHR vendor and device vendors for interface development or middleware*
Is bidirectional interface in place (orders & results)?	Full bidirectional	Results only	No interface	*Implement ADT and order feeds from EHR to devices; validate result return*
Are all devices registered in device management system?	100% registered	Partially registered	No system	*Implement medical device management (MDM) system; register and track all devices*
Is device data quality monitored continuously?	Automated monitoring	Manual spot-checks	No monitoring	*Implement interface monitoring dashboard; define data quality SLAs with IT team*
Have staff been trained on device digital workflows?	All staff trained	Some training done	No training	*Build device-specific digital workflow training into competency programs for all roles*

Is downtime procedure defined for device failures?	Written, tested protocol	Informal procedure	No procedure	*Write and test downtime procedures for every critical device type; include in disaster recovery plan*

USA vs. India: Equipment Digitization Context

The equipment digitization challenge looks different in the United States and India; but it is equally urgent in both contexts, for different reasons.

United States	India
Situation: Equipment is largely digital but often poorly integrated • Most clinical devices have digital output, the hardware problem is largely solved • The challenge is integration: many devices still not connected to EHR: nurses manually transcribe from device to screen • Legacy equipment (10-20 years old) may have digital output but use obsolete protocols, middleware solutions or replacement needed • IoT medical devices (wearables, remote monitors) proliferating, integration governance critical • **Action: Conduct device integration audit; prioritize high-volume, high-risk devices first (ICU monitors, infusion pumps, lab analyzers)**	**Situation: Equipment mix ranges from world-class to basic analog** • Leading private hospitals (Apollo, Fortis, Manipal) have modern digital equipment comparable to US standards • Mid-tier private hospitals: mixed, newer wards may be digital, older units still analog • Government hospitals: significant proportion of equipment still analog or basic digital without integration capability • Opportunity: New hospital builds should specify digital-first equipment procurement, no analog equipment purchased after 2024 • **Action: Equipment digitization as capital investment phase, build the business case around error reduction, staff time savings, and AI readiness**

Paperless as the Great Milestone: What It Truly Means

When a hospital achieves true paperless operations, not just paperless on paper, but genuinely, verifiably paperless in every clinical workflow, it deserves to celebrate. Because it means something profound has been accomplished.

It means that every vital sign, every medication, every laboratory result, every physician order, every nursing assessment, every imaging study, and every clinical note exists in a single digital record: accurate, timestamped, attributable, accessible, and analyzable. It means that a physician can review a patient's complete history from any terminal in the hospital. It means that an AI system has access to the complete picture it needs to generate reliable predictions. It means that quality measurement is automatic, not manual. It means that data moves at the speed of care.

This milestone is not about eliminating paper as a material. It is about eliminating the disconnection, delay, error, and opacity that paper represents. A truly paperless hospital is a transparent hospital, one where clinical practice can be seen, measured, improved, and trusted.

The Five Markers of True Paperless Achievement

- Marker 1, Zero manual transcription: No clinical data is manually re-entered from a device, paper, or verbal report into a digital system. All data flows are automated and verified
- Marker 2, Complete digital medication cycle: Prescribing, verification, dispensing, administration, and reconciliation are all electronic, barcode-verified, and EHR-documented without exception
- Marker 3, Real-time clinical documentation: All physician orders, nursing notes, and clinical assessments are documented digitally at the point of care, within the same encounter, not retrospectively
- Marker 4, Electronic results delivery: All laboratory results, radiology reports, and diagnostic findings are delivered to ordering clinicians electronically, with auto-filing to the patient record and critical value alerting

- Marker 5, Auditable data trail: Every data entry, modification, access, and transmission is logged with user ID, timestamp, and device ID, creating a complete, tamper-evident audit trail for every patient record

Building the Business Case for Equipment Digitization

For hospital boards, finance committees, and senior leadership, particularly in India, where capital investment decisions require compelling justification, the equipment digitization investment must be framed as a business case, not just a technology aspiration.

- Patient safety ROI: studies consistently show that automated data collection reduces medication errors by 50-80% and critical value reporting delays by 60-90%, costs that are measurable in adverse events avoided, liability reduced, and accreditation maintained
- Staff efficiency: nurses in manual-transcription environments spend an average of 25-35% of their shift on documentation. Automated data collection reclaims that time for direct patient care, the highest-value use of nursing hours
- Data quality for AI: every percentage point improvement in data completeness and accuracy translates directly to AI model performance, and AI ROI depends entirely on data quality
- Accreditation requirement: NABH (India) and Joint Commission (USA) accreditation standards increasingly require electronic documentation and medication administration verification, equipment digitization is not optional for accredited facilities
- Competitive differentiation: in markets where patients have choice, digital capability is increasingly a factor in provider selection, particularly among educated, urban patient populations in both the USA and India

7.3 The Paperless Hospital: Why It Is Essential and How to Get There

A paperless hospital is not a luxury. It is a patient safety imperative. Paper-based systems, handwritten medication orders, paper clinical notes, manual lab result transcription, physical file transport, are inherently error-prone, difficult to audit, impossible to analyze at scale, and inaccessible to AI.

Every hour that a clinical note exists only on paper is an hour during which that information cannot trigger an AI alert, cannot be accessed by a covering physician at 2 AM, cannot be analyzed for quality improvement, and cannot follow the patient to another provider. Paper is not just inefficient, it is dangerous.

The Paperless Transition: A Phased Approach

Transitioning from paper to fully digital operations requires a structured, phased approach. Attempting to digitize everything simultaneously, a common and costly mistake, typically leads to partial implementation, frustrated staff, and a retreat to paper for critical functions.

Phase 1	FOUNDATION: Implement core EHR with patient registration, demographic management, and basic clinical documentation. Digitize medication orders, laboratory result delivery, and appointment scheduling. Establish network infrastructure and hardware. Train all staff on EHR basics. Timeline: 6-12 months.
Phase 2	CLINICAL INTEGRATION: Expand EHR to full clinical documentation across all departments, nursing notes, physician orders, operative records, discharge summaries. Integrate laboratory, radiology, and pharmacy systems. Implement clinical decision support alerts. Begin structured data capture for quality metrics. Timeline: 12-24 months.
Phase 3	INTELLIGENCE: Activate AI tools using the clean, integrated data now available. Deploy predictive analytics, automated quality monitoring, and administrative optimization systems.

	Achieve full interoperability with external providers. Begin population health management. Timeline: 24-48 months.
Phase 4	OPTIMIZATION: Continuous improvement of digital systems based on data and feedback. Advanced AI applications. Patient-facing digital engagement. Community health integration. Research data infrastructure. Ongoing.

7.4 Cloud-Based Healthcare Platforms

The shift to cloud-based healthcare platforms is one of the most significant infrastructure changes in hospital digital transformation. Cloud computing offers healthcare organizations access to virtually unlimited storage, powerful computing resources, and sophisticated software applications, without the capital expense and maintenance burden of on-premise server infrastructure.

Benefits of Cloud in Healthcare

- Scalability: cloud infrastructure scales instantly with demand, critical for hospitals with seasonal census variation or AI workloads that require significant computing power for model training
- Cost efficiency: operational expense model replaces large capital investments, particularly important for healthcare organizations in India, where capital is constrained
- Reliability: major cloud providers (AWS, Microsoft Azure, Google Cloud) offer service availability guarantees that exceed what most hospitals can achieve with on-premise infrastructure
- AI access: cloud platforms provide access to pre-built AI services, medical imaging APIs, NLP services, predictive analytics tools; that would be prohibitively expensive to build independently
- Disaster recovery: cloud-based data is backed up across multiple geographic locations: critical for business continuity in the event of a natural disaster, cyber attack, or equipment failure

Cloud Security and Compliance Requirements

Healthcare data is among the most sensitive personal information that exists, and cloud storage of patient data requires rigorous security measures and regulatory compliance. In the United States, cloud vendors must be HIPAA-compliant and must sign a Business Associate Agreement (BAA) with the healthcare organization. HITRUST certification provides additional assurance of security controls.

In India, the Digital Personal Data Protection Act (DPDPA) 2023 establishes requirements for patient data privacy and security, including data localization requirements that affect cloud provider selection. Healthcare organizations must ensure that cloud vendors hosting patient data are compliant with applicable Indian regulations.

Both USA and India contexts require encryption of data in transit and at rest, robust access controls and audit trails, regular security assessments, and vendor due diligence that goes beyond price comparison.

7.5 Interoperability: Making the Digital Hospital Communicate

A hospital that has digitized its own operations but cannot share data with other providers, payers, and public health systems has completed only half of the transformation. Interoperability, the ability of different health information systems to exchange and use data meaningfully, is the capability that transforms a digital hospital into a connected healthcare ecosystem.

The Interoperability Standards Healthcare Leaders Must Know

- HL7 v2: the most widely deployed healthcare messaging standard, used for transmitting lab results, ADT (admission/discharge/transfer) data, and orders between systems
- HL7 FHIR (Fast Healthcare Interoperability Resources): the modern standard for health data exchange, uses web APIs, required by the 21st Century Cures Act in the USA, adopted by NDHM in India

- DICOM (Digital Imaging and Communications in Medicine): the universal standard for medical imaging data, essential for radiology AI integration
- ICD-10: the international standard for diagnosis coding, used for clinical documentation, billing, quality measurement, and AI training data
- SNOMED CT: a comprehensive clinical terminology system, used for standardized representation of clinical concepts in EHR systems
- LOINC (Logical Observation Identifiers Names and Codes): the standard for laboratory and clinical observation codes, essential for clean, analyzable laboratory data

For hospital leaders, the practical implication of these standards is simple but non-negotiable: every technology system you purchase must support these standards. Vendor contracts must specify conformance requirements. Your technology team must verify conformance before go-live. And your data governance framework must include monitoring of data exchange quality to ensure that interoperability works as intended, not just in the vendor demonstration, but in daily clinical operations.

7.6 Cybersecurity in Healthcare: The Non-Negotiable Imperative

Healthcare is the most targeted sector for cyberattacks globally. In 2023, the healthcare industry experienced more data breaches than any other sector in the United States. Ransomware attacks on hospitals have resulted in patient deaths, through diverted ambulances, delayed surgeries, and unavailable medication records. In India, multiple major hospital chains have experienced significant cyber incidents in recent years.

For healthcare leaders, cybersecurity is not an IT budget line item. It is a patient safety issue, and a legal, financial, and reputational risk of the first order. The digital hospital is only as valuable as it is secure.

The Healthcare Cybersecurity Framework

The US National Institute of Standards and Technology (NIST) Cybersecurity Framework provides the most widely used structure for healthcare security management: Identify, Protect, Detect, Respond, and Recover. This framework applies equally in India, where CERT-In (Computer Emergency Response Team, India) provides guidance on cybersecurity standards for critical infrastructure, including healthcare.

Preventive Controls	Detection & Monitoring	Response & Recovery
• Multi-factor authentication for all systems • Role-based access control, minimum necessary access • Encryption of all patient data at rest and in transit • Regular security patches and updates, zero tolerance for known vulnerabilities • Staff phishing awareness training, the human firewall • Vendor security assessment for all third-party systems	• 24/7 Security Operations Center (SOC) monitoring • Network anomaly detection, AI-powered threat identification • EHR access audit trails, automated alerts for suspicious access patterns • Medical device security monitoring, IoT devices are a major vulnerability • Regular penetration testing, testing your own defenses • Threat intelligence feeds, awareness of	• Documented Incident Response Plan, tested annually • Ransomware-specific response protocol • Offline data backups, tested regularly for restoration capability • Business continuity plan for downtime procedures • Regulatory breach notification, HIPAA (72 hrs, USA), CERT-In (6 hrs, India) • Post-incident review and improvement process

	emerging attack vectors	

The Human Element: Training as the First Line of Defense

More than 90% of successful cyberattacks begin with human error, a phishing email opened, a password shared, a USB drive plugged in. Technology controls are essential, but the human firewall is the most important and most frequently neglected layer of cybersecurity.

Every staff member in a digital hospital must receive cybersecurity awareness training, not once at onboarding, but regularly and continuously. Simulated phishing exercises test and reinforce vigilance. Clear policies and easy reporting mechanisms for suspicious activity encourage a security culture. And leadership must model the behaviors it expects: using strong passwords, logging out of systems when not in use, and following security protocols even when they are inconvenient.

In both USA and India, cybersecurity training requirements are increasingly part of accreditation standards. The Joint Commission and NABH both include information security in their assessment frameworks. For world-class hospitals, this is not a compliance exercise; it is a patient safety culture element.

7.7 Patient-Facing Digital Engagement

Digital transformation is not only about internal hospital systems. World-class digital hospitals also invest in patient-facing digital capabilities that extend care beyond the hospital walls, empower patients to manage their own health, and improve the care experience.

Patient-Facing Digital Capabilities, From Basic to Advanced
• Patient portal: secure online access to health records, lab results, appointment scheduling, and secure messaging with the care team, standard of care in the USA, rapidly growing in India • Telemedicine: video consultation with physicians, expanded dramatically during COVID-19, now a permanent feature of

world-class care delivery for follow-up visits and chronic disease management

- Mobile health apps: condition-specific apps for diabetes management, hypertension monitoring, medication adherence, connected to EHR for clinical visibility
- Remote patient monitoring: wearable devices and home monitoring equipment that transmit continuous data to the care team, enabling proactive intervention before hospital visits
- AI-powered symptom checkers: intelligent triage tools that help patients determine when and where to seek care, reducing unnecessary ED visits and improving appropriate care utilization
- Automated follow-up: AI-generated post-discharge messages, appointment reminders, and medication adherence support, reducing readmission rates by maintaining care continuity

7.8 Real-World Reflection: Digital Transformation Leadership Lessons

Across thirty years of organizational consulting, in manufacturing, technology, and now healthcare, the patterns of successful and failed digital transformations are remarkably consistent. The lessons apply whether you are leading a 50-bed community hospital in Gujarat or a 500-bed tertiary care center in Texas.

- **Lesson 1, Start with why, not what: The most successful transformations begin with a clear articulation of how digital systems will improve patient care and staff experience, not with a technology selection process. When people understand why the change is happening, they are far more likely to support how it is implemented.**

- **Lesson 2, Involve frontline staff from day one: Clinical staff who are involved in system selection, workflow design, and testing are champions at go-live. Those who learn about the new system on the day it goes live are resistors. There is no shortcut to this engagement, and no more costly mistake than bypassing it.**

- **Lesson 3, Train beyond the system: Training for digital transformation must go beyond how to use the software. It must address why the system works the way it does, how to handle downtime procedures, and how to maintain quality of care during the transition period when workflows are still adjusting.**

- **Lesson 4, Measure everything, from the beginning: Define your baseline metrics before go-live, patient wait times, documentation completion rates, medication error rates, staff satisfaction. Track them throughout implementation. This data demonstrates value, identifies problems early, and supports the business case for continued investment.**

- **Lesson 5, Celebrate progress, address problems quickly: Digital transformation is a multi-year journey with setbacks as**

well as advances. Leaders who celebrate genuine milestones build momentum. Leaders who address problems transparently and quickly, rather than minimizing them, build the trust that sustains long change journeys.

★ KEY TAKEAWAYS

15. Digital transformation is fundamentally a people and culture project, technology is the tool, leadership is the driver.
16. Paperless hospital operations are a patient safety imperative: paper-based systems are error-prone, unauditable, and incompatible with AI.
17. The four phases of digital transformation: Foundation, Clinical Integration, Intelligence, and Optimization, must be sequenced thoughtfully, not rushed.
18. Cloud-based platforms offer scalability, cost efficiency, and AI access, but require rigorous security compliance with HIPAA (USA) and DPDPA (India).
19. Interoperability via HL7 FHIR is non-negotiable: every system purchased must support open data exchange standards.
20. Cybersecurity is a patient safety issue: Ransomware can kill. Prevention requires both technical controls and continuous staff training.
21. Patient-facing digital capabilities, portals, telemedicine, remote monitoring, extend world-class care beyond the hospital walls.
22. Five leadership lessons: start with why, involve frontline staff early, train beyond the system, measure everything, celebrate progress, and address problems quickly.

▶ COMING NEXT

Part 3 of this book moves from technology to quality, from the digital systems that collect and analyze data to the quality management frameworks that make improvement systematic, sustainable, and patient-centered. Chapter 8 begins with the definition, principles, and measurement of quality in healthcare.

PART THREE

Quality, Excellence & Systems Thinking

Building healthcare systems that are consistent, safe, measurable, and always improving

Chapter 8

Quality in Healthcare

What It Means, Why It Matters, and How to Build It Into Every System and Every Person

> *"Quality is not an act. It is a habit."*
>
> **Aristotle whose insight, 2,400 years later, remains the most precise definition of what quality culture requires.**

8.1 Introduction: Quality Is the Foundation of Everything

Every chapter in this book, on AI, on digital systems, on data governance, on medical education, ultimately serves one purpose: to improve the quality of healthcare delivered to patients. Quality is not a department. It is not a checklist. It is not what happens when an accreditation survey is scheduled. Quality is the operating standard of a world-class healthcare institution, embedded in every process, every decision, every interaction, and every person.

This chapter defines quality in healthcare with precision, examines the dimensions by which it must be measured, explores the most important patient safety frameworks developed in the United States and India, and builds the foundation for the quality management tools and AI integration approaches described in Chapters 9 and 10.

For leaders with backgrounds in manufacturing or service industries, much of this chapter will feel familiar, and intentionally so. The principles of quality are universal. What makes a Toyota factory excellent is structurally similar to what makes a hospital excellent. The specific tools, the regulatory environment, and the human stakes are different. But the underlying logic, define quality, measure it, find the gaps, fix the root cause, prevent recurrence, and improve again, is the same logic that drives excellence in every domain.

8.2 Defining Quality in Healthcare: A Multi-Dimensional Framework

Quality in healthcare is not a single concept. It is a framework of interconnected dimensions, each of which must be actively managed for an organization to deliver truly excellent care. The most widely accepted framework, developed by the Institute of Medicine (IOM) in the United States and adopted globally, defines quality healthcare as care that is:

	Dimension	What It Means in Practice
1	**SAFE** No harm from care itself, preventing errors, infections, falls, and adverse events	AI early warning systems, clinical decision support, barcode medication administration, automated safety alerts
2	**EFFECTIVE** Evidence-based care that achieves the intended outcomes, right treatment, right patient	AI diagnostic support, protocol adherence monitoring, outcome tracking, comparative effectiveness analytics
3	**PATIENT-CENTERED** Care that respects patient preferences, values, and dignity, the patient is a partner	AI-generated personalized care plans, patient portal engagement, automated preference capture in EHR
4	**TIMELY** Reducing harmful delays in care delivery, for patients and for clinical staff	AI scheduling optimization, predictive census management, automated result delivery, real-time triage support
5	**EFFICIENT** Avoiding waste, of time, equipment, medications, energy, and human effort	Lean AI-powered workflow optimization, predictive supply management, automated documentation
6	**EQUITABLE** The same quality of care regardless of race, gender, income, language, or geography	AI bias monitoring, population health analytics, and remote monitoring for underserved populations

These six dimensions are not independent; they are deeply interconnected. A care system that is efficient but not safe is failing. One that is effective but not equitable is delivering excellence to some patients and mediocrity to others. A system that is patient-centered but not timely frustrates the very patients it claims to respect. World-class quality requires all six dimensions, measured continuously, and improved systematically.

8.3 Patient Safety: The Non-Negotiable Core

Of all the dimensions of healthcare quality, patient safety is the most fundamental. It is the condition on which every other dimension depends. A healthcare system that harms its patients, through preventable errors, infections, falls, medication mistakes, or diagnostic failures, has failed at its most basic responsibility, regardless of what its patient satisfaction scores or efficiency metrics show.

The scale of the patient safety problem is sobering. The landmark Institute of Medicine report 'To Err is Human' (1999) estimated that medical errors cause between 44,000 and 98,000 deaths annually in the United States. Subsequent research has placed the true figure higher, with some estimates suggesting that preventable medical errors are the third leading cause of death in the US. In India, a country with 1.4 billion people and a healthcare system serving enormous volumes, the absolute numbers of preventable harm events are significant, though comprehensive national data collection remains a work in progress.

The global patient safety movement has produced a powerful body of knowledge, tools, and frameworks over the past 25 years. Every hospital leader, in Houston or in Kadi, must be fluent in this knowledge, because it is the foundation on which all other quality improvement work is built.

The Swiss Cheese Model: Understanding How Errors Happen

The most important conceptual model in patient safety is James Reason's Swiss Cheese Model. It teaches us that serious adverse events in healthcare almost never result from a single failure by a single person. They result from the simultaneous alignment of multiple small failures:

like holes in Swiss cheese lining up so that a hazard can pass through every defensive layer.

In a medication error, for example, the prescriber writes an unclear order (hole 1). The pharmacist does not catch the ambiguity (hole 2). The nurse administering the medication is interrupted and does not complete the five rights check (hole 3). The bedside barcode scanner is malfunctioning (hole 4). The patient receives the wrong dose. No single person is solely responsible. The system failed.

This model has a profound implication for quality leadership: the response to an adverse event must never begin with blame. It must begin with system analysis. What holes were present? Which defenses failed? What needs to be fixed so that the alignment cannot occur again? This is the difference between a blaming culture, which drives errors underground and prevents learning, and a safety culture, which surfaces errors, analyzes them honestly, and continuously strengthens the system's defenses.

Building a Patient Safety Culture, The Seven Requirements

- Leadership commitment: senior leaders visibly and consistently prioritize safety over production pressure; the tone at the top sets the culture throughout. Psychological safety: every staff member, from the surgeon to the ward aide, feels safe to report errors, near-misses, and concerns without fear of punishment or humiliation
- Blame-free reporting systems: incident reporting is easy, anonymous where needed, and responded to with learning rather than discipline
- Root Cause Analysis (RCA): every serious adverse event triggers a systematic investigation of contributing factors, not a search for who to blame
- Transparency: patient safety data is shared openly with staff, leadership, and, where appropriate, patients and families.
- Standardization: evidence-based protocols, checklists, and bundles reduce reliance on individual memory and judgment for high-risk tasks

- Measurement: patient safety indicators are tracked continuously, reviewed regularly, and used to drive improvement, not just to satisfy accreditors

High-Reliability Organizations (HRO): The Gold Standard for Healthcare

High-Reliability Organizations (HROs) are institutions that operate in high-risk, complex environments such as nuclear power plants, aircraft carriers, commercial aviation, and achieve extraordinarily low rates of catastrophic failure over long periods of time. Healthcare has adopted the HRO framework as the model for world-class patient safety.

HROs share five defining characteristics that translate directly to healthcare: preoccupation with failure (always looking for what could go wrong, not just what went wrong), reluctance to simplify (resisting the temptation to explain complex problems with simple causes), sensitivity to operations (leadership staying close to the front line, aware of what is actually happening), commitment to resilience (building the capacity to detect, contain, and recover from errors before they cause harm), and deference to expertise (deferring to the most knowledgeable person, regardless of hierarchy, in time-critical situations).

Applying HRO principles in Indian and American hospitals requires cultural work as well as system work. In both contexts, hierarchical cultures can suppress the reporting and the 'speaking up' that safety requires. Medical education that rewards certainty over intellectual humility can create the kind of overconfidence safety experts consider one of the most dangerous conditions in high-risk systems.

8.4 Error Reduction: Tools and Techniques That Save Lives

Patient safety culture creates the conditions for error reduction. But culture alone is not enough, specific tools and techniques must be implemented to systematically reduce the frequency and severity of clinical errors.

Checklists & Bundles	SBAR & Communication	Technology Safeguards
• Surgical Safety Checklist (WHO), reduces surgical mortality by 47% in studies • Central Line Bundle: 5-element protocol eliminates most CLABSIs • VAP Bundle, ventilator-associated pneumonia prevention • Sepsis Bundle (Hour-1 Bundle), time-critical interventions for sepsis • Medication Reconciliation Checklist, on admission, transfer, discharge	• SBAR (Situation-Background-Assessment-Recommendation), structured handoff communication • Read-back and verification for verbal orders, prevents mishearing errors • Standardized handoff protocols, I-PASS, SIGNOUT • Closed-loop communication in codes and rapid response • Structured family communication, reduces adverse events from information gaps • TeamSTEPPS, team training for high-reliability communication	• Barcode Medication Administration (BCMA), verifies 5 rights at point of care • Computerized Physician Order Entry (CPOE), eliminates handwriting errors • Drug interaction and allergy alerts in EHR/CDSS • Smart infusion pumps with drug libraries, prevents dosing errors • Patient identification wristbands with barcode, prevents wrong-patient events • AI early warning

• Daily ICU Goals Checklist, aligns entire team on patient priorities		systems: sepsis, deterioration, fall risk prediction

8.5 Continuous Improvement: The Operating Philosophy of Excellence

Patient safety addresses what goes wrong. Continuous improvement addresses how everything can become better, even when nothing has gone obviously wrong. World-class healthcare institutions do not wait for adverse events to drive change. They continuously examine their processes, measure their performance, compare themselves to the best in the world, and relentlessly pursue better.

The philosophical foundation of continuous improvement in healthcare is the same as in manufacturing, and it was articulated most powerfully by W. Edwards Deming, whose 14 Points of Management and System of Profound Knowledge transformed Japanese industry after World War II and subsequently transformed quality thinking in every sector, including healthcare.

Deming's most important insight for healthcare leaders is this: 94% of problems in any organization are caused by the systems, not by the people working within them. This means that when a nurse makes a medication error, when a patient waits four hours in an emergency department, or when an operating case is cancelled for preventable reasons, the correct response is not to blame the individual, but to examine and improve the system that produced that outcome. This is not an excuse for individual accountability; it is a reorientation of leadership energy toward the place where most leverage exists: system design.

8.6 Measuring Quality: Key Performance Indicators for Healthcare

What cannot be measured cannot be managed and what cannot be managed cannot be improved. This is perhaps the single most important practical principle in quality management, and it applies to healthcare with particular force, because the outcomes being measured are human lives, health, and dignity.

A world-class healthcare quality measurement system tracks indicators across three categories: structural measures (what resources and capabilities exist), process measures (what care is being delivered), and outcome measures (what results are being achieved for patients). All three are necessary: none is sufficient alone.

< 2%	< 1%	> 95%	< 30d
Hospital-Acquired Infection Rate Target	Surgical Mortality Rate Benchmark	Medication Administration Accuracy Target	Readmission Rate Monitoring Window

Essential Quality KPIs Every Hospital Must Track, USA and India

- PATIENT SAFETY: Hospital-Acquired Infection (HAI) rates by type (CLABSI, CAUTI, SSI, VAP); medication error rate; patient fall rate with injury; pressure injury prevalence; wrong-site surgery rate
- CLINICAL EFFECTIVENESS: Adherence to evidence-based care bundles (sepsis, AMI, stroke, pneumonia); readmission rates by diagnosis; mortality rates (observed vs. expected); surgical complication rates
- TIMELINESS: ED door-to-physician time; door-to-balloon time for STEMI; time to antibiotic for sepsis; elective surgery wait times; discharge time of day distribution
- PATIENT EXPERIENCE: Patient satisfaction scores (HCAHPS in USA; NABH patient feedback in India); complaint volume and resolution time; informed consent completeness; communication effectiveness ratings
- EFFICIENCY: Average length of stay by DRG/diagnosis; operating theatre utilization rate; bed occupancy rate; supply cost per case; staff overtime percentage
- WORKFORCE: Staff turnover rate by department; training completion rates; incident report submission rate; safety huddle participation rate; AI system utilization rates post-implementation

8.7 Quality Standards and Accreditation: USA and India

Healthcare accreditation is the external validation that an institution meets defined quality and safety standards. It serves both as a quality improvement mechanism because the preparation process drives genuine improvement and as a credibility signal. signal to patients, payers, and the community. Every world-class hospital in both the United States and India pursues and maintains accreditation.

Country	Accreditation Body / Standard	Key Quality Focus Areas
USA	The Joint Commission (TJC), hospital accreditation standard; recognized by CMS for Medicare/Medicaid participation	National Patient Safety Goals; medication management; infection control; surgical safety; patient rights; leadership standards; emergency management
USA	Centers for Medicare & Medicaid Services (CMS), Conditions of Participation; required for all Medicare/Medicaid-participating hospitals	Quality reporting (IPPS, VBP program); star ratings; readmission penalties; HAC reduction; patient experience (HCAHPS) scores
USA	DNV Healthcare / HFAP / NIAHO, alternative CMS-approved accreditation bodies with ISO-based standards	ISO 9001-aligned quality management system integration; continuous survey process rather than periodic survey
India	NABH (National Accreditation Board for Hospitals & Healthcare Providers), the gold standard for Indian hospital accreditation	Patient-centered care; patient safety; clinical care standards; infection control; quality improvement; human resource management; facility management
India	JCI (Joint Commission International), international accreditation pursued by leading Indian private hospitals	Equivalent to US Joint Commission standards; recognized by international payers and medical tourism patients; highest global benchmark
Global	ISO 9001:2015, Quality Management System standard	Process documentation; customer (patient) focus; risk-based thinking; continual improvement; leadership

	applicable to healthcare organizations	commitment; evidence-based decision-making
Global	ISO 15189, Medical Laboratory Quality and Competence standard	Specific to clinical laboratories; technical competence; management requirements; traceability; uncertainty of measurement

★ KEY TAKEAWAYS

1. Quality in healthcare has six dimensions: Safe, Effective, Patient-Centered, Timely, Efficient, and Equitable, all must be managed simultaneously.
2. Patient safety is the non-negotiable foundation: the Swiss Cheese Model teaches us that errors are system failures, not individual failures, the response is system improvement, not blame.
3. High-Reliability Organization (HRO) principles, preoccupation with failure, sensitivity to operations, deference to expertise, are the gold standard for healthcare safety culture.
4. Specific error-reduction tools, checklists, SBAR, BCMA, CPOE, AI early warning, must be implemented systematically, not selectively.
5. Measurement is mandatory: quality KPIs across safety, effectiveness, timeliness, experience, efficiency, and workforce must be tracked continuously and reviewed at every level.
6. Accreditation (Joint Commission/CMS in USA; NABH/JCI in India) is the minimum standard, world-class institutions continuously exceed it.
7. Quality culture begins at the top and lives on the front line: it requires daily habits, psychological safety, transparent data, and leaders who model the behaviors they expect.

▶ COMING NEXT

Chapter 9 introduces the most powerful systematic improvement methodology in healthcare: Lean Six Sigma. You will learn how waste elimination and variance reduction, proven in manufacturing, translate directly into better patient care, shorter wait times, fewer errors, and more efficient operations.

Chapter 9

Lean Six Sigma in Healthcare

Eliminating Waste, Reducing Variation, and Building a Culture of Systematic Improvement

> *"If you can't describe what you are doing as a process, you don't know what you're doing."*
>
> **W. Edwards Deming whose process thinking is the foundation of every Lean and Six Sigma methodology in this chapter.**

9.1 Introduction: Why Lean Six Sigma Belongs in Every Hospital

Lean and Six Sigma were developed in manufacturing, Lean in Toyota's production system in Japan, Six Sigma at Motorola and General Electric in the United States. Both methodologies were refined over decades to solve problems that are endemic to healthcare: wasted time, inconsistent processes, preventable defects, and systems that depend too heavily on individual heroics rather than reliable design.

The application of Lean Six Sigma to healthcare is no longer experimental. It is proven. The Virginia Mason Medical Center in Seattle transformed itself using the Toyota Production System, reducing patient wait times, eliminating millions of dollars of waste, and dramatically improving patient safety outcomes. The Cleveland Clinic, Mayo Clinic, and ThedaCare in the United States have all used Lean Six Sigma to achieve measurable, sustained quality improvements. In India, leading hospitals including Apollo, Narayana Health (which Dr. Devi Shetty built explicitly on manufacturing quality principles), and Fortis have applied Lean principles to achieve cost and quality breakthroughs that serve as global benchmarks.

This chapter gives healthcare leaders the practical knowledge to understand, champion, and lead Lean Six Sigma initiatives: and to connect these improvement methodologies directly to AI implementation for the next generation of quality management.

9.2 Understanding Lean: The Science of Waste Elimination

Lean is a management philosophy and a set of practical tools focused on identifying and eliminating waste, any activity that consumes resources without adding value for the patient. In manufacturing, waste means defective products, excess inventory, unnecessary movement, and waiting time. In healthcare, waste means patients waiting, staff searching for supplies, duplicate documentation, unnecessary tests, and processes that consume time and resources without improving care.

The starting point for Lean thinking is the identification of value from the patient's perspective. Every activity in a healthcare process is either value-adding (the patient would pay for it, a skilled procedure, a clinical assessment, a medication that treats their condition) or non-value-adding (Patients wait, staff re-enter data already captured, the specimen sits in transit). Lean methodology relentlessly targets the non-value-adding activities.

The Eight Wastes in Healthcare: TIMWOODS

The eight categories of waste in Lean, remembered by the acronym TIMWOODS, provide a systematic framework for identifying improvement opportunities in any healthcare process. Each waste type has specific manifestations in clinical and operational settings that every healthcare leader should be able to recognize.

Waste Type	Definition	Healthcare Example	Elimination Strategy
T, Transport	Unnecessary movement of patients, specimens, medications, or information	Patient transported twice for the same imaging study; specimens sent to wrong lab then re-sent; paper records physically carried between departments	Redesign patient flow; implement pneumatic tube systems; digitize information transport; map physical layout against patient journey
I, Inventory	Excess supplies, medications, or equipment beyond immediate need	Overstocked medication carts leading to expiry waste; excess surgical supplies in ORs; unused single-use device inventory	Just-in-time supply management; AI-powered inventory forecasting; consignment models with vendors; par level management
M, Motion	Unnecessary movement of staff during care delivery	Nurses walking long distances to retrieve supplies stored away from point of care; physicians navigating multiple systems to find patient information	5S workplace organization; decentralized supply storage at point of care; unified EHR with single sign-on; workstation-on-wheels
W, Waiting	Patients, staff, or information waiting idle at any stage of care	ED patients waiting 4 hours for admission bed; results waiting in system before clinician notification; OR cases delayed for equipment sterilization	Pull systems for bed management; AI-powered result alerting; predictive scheduling; STAT specimen protocols

O, Overproduction	Doing more than the patient needs, excess tests, documentation, or steps	Routine daily labs ordered by habit without clinical indication; duplicate documentation in paper and digital; unnecessary specialist consultations	Evidence-based order sets with clinical criteria; duplicate documentation elimination; clinical indication requirements for high-cost tests
O, Overprocessing	More steps or complexity in a process than necessary for the outcome	Multiple approval signatures for routine orders; lengthy paper consent forms for minor procedures; redundant safety checks that duplicate each other	Process mapping to identify redundant steps; standardized consent processes; electronic signature with single verification
D, Defects	Errors that require correction, rework, or cause harm	Medication errors requiring intervention; specimen labelling errors causing re-collection; incorrect coding requiring claims reprocessing	Barcode verification at every point; standard operating procedures; error-proofing (poka-yoke); root cause analysis for every defect
S, Skills	Underutilizing the talent, knowledge, and capability of staff	Physicians performing tasks within nurse scope; nurses performing tasks within aide scope; quality data analyzed by consultants rather than front-line staff	Scope of practice optimization; staff empowerment in improvement projects; training staff as quality champions;

			suggestion systems with response

9.3 Lean Tools in Healthcare: The Practical Toolkit

Lean thinking becomes Lean practice through a set of specific tools and techniques. Each tool has proven applications in healthcare settings, in the United States and in India.

Value Stream Mapping (VSM)

Value Stream Mapping is Lean's most powerful diagnostic tool. It creates a visual map of every step in a patient's journey through a process, from entry to exit, showing where time is spent, where waiting occurs, where handoffs happen, and where value is added versus wasted. A VSM of the ED patient journey, for example, typically reveals that the vast majority of time a patient spends in the ED is waiting, waiting for triage, waiting for a physician, waiting for test results, waiting for a decision, waiting for a bed. The actual clinical care time is often a small fraction of total ED time.

Creating a VSM requires walking the actual process with the people who work in it: observing, timing, mapping, and questioning. The current-state map reveals process inefficiencies and delays. The future-state map, designed by the improvement team, shows what the process should look like when waste is eliminated. The gap between them defines the improvement work.

5S: Workplace Organization

5S is a systematic approach to workplace organization: Sort (remove everything not needed), Set in Order (organize what remains for maximum efficiency), Shine (clean and maintain), Standardize (document the organized state as the standard), and Sustain (build habits and audits to maintain it). In healthcare, 5S applied to a medication room, a nursing station, or a procedure cart reduces the time staff spend searching for supplies, reduces the risk of using expired or wrong items, and creates a cleaner, safer environment for both staff and patients.

5S is often the entry point for Lean in healthcare because its results are immediate, visible, and universally valued by front-line staff. A nursing station transformed by 5S is one where every item has a designated, labeled place, and where staff can tell at a glance whether something is missing or out of place. This visual management creates the environmental foundation for everything else that Lean requires.

Kaizen: Continuous Small Improvements

Kaizen is the Japanese concept of continuous improvement, small, incremental changes made continuously by the people closest to the work. Unlike large restructuring projects, Kaizen operates at the level of daily practice: a nurse identifies a more efficient way to set up a wound care kit; a pharmacist redesigns the medication dispensing workflow to eliminate one unnecessary step; a registration clerk creates a simple visual cue that reduces patient information errors.

The power of Kaizen is not in any individual improvement; it is in the culture it creates. An organization where every person, every day, is looking for small ways to improve is an organization that compounds improvement over time into extraordinary performance. In healthcare, Kaizen events (structured 3-5 day improvement workshops focused on a specific process) can produce dramatic results in short timeframes, reducing patient wait times by 30-50%, reducing supply costs by 20-30%, and improving staff satisfaction by making their work less frustrating.

9.4 Understanding Six Sigma: The Science of Variance Reduction

While Lean focuses on eliminating waste and improving flow, Six Sigma focuses on reducing variance: the unpredictable variation in process outputs that leads to defects, errors, and inconsistent results. In healthcare, variance kills. When a sepsis bundle is applied consistently 100% of the time, mortality falls. When it is applied inconsistently, 70% of the time, with varying elements, outcomes are unpredictable, and avoidable deaths occur.

Six Sigma takes its name from the statistical concept of standard deviation (sigma). A process operating at Six Sigma quality produces only 3.4 defects per million opportunities, an extraordinarily low defect rate. Most healthcare processes operate far below this standard. The goal of Six Sigma is not necessarily to reach 3.4 defects per million in every process; it is to apply statistical rigor to understanding, measuring, and reducing variation wherever it causes harm.

DMAIC: The Six Sigma Improvement Framework

The core methodology of Six Sigma improvement is DMAIC: Define, Measure, Analyze, Improve, Control. This structured problem-solving framework ensures that improvement is based on data, not assumptions, and that solutions address root causes rather than symptoms.

Phase	What It Means	Healthcare Application	Key Tools
D Define	Define the problem, the goal, the scope, and the impact on patients. Write a clear problem statement and project charter.	Define: 'ED patients with sepsis are receiving first antibiotic more than 3 hours after triage. Goal: achieve < 1 hour in 90% of cases.'	Project Charter; SIPOC diagram; Voice of the Customer (patient feedback); problem statement template
M Measure	Collect baseline data to quantify the current state. Validate measurement systems. Establish the performance baseline.	Measure antibiotic time from EHR data for past 6 months. Baseline: median 210 minutes. Only 28% of cases under 60 minutes. Data validated.	Process mapping; data collection plan; measurement system analysis (MSA); control charts; Pareto charts; histogram
A Analyze	Identify root causes of the problem using	Root causes identified: sepsis screening not done at	Fishbone (Ishikawa) diagram; 5-Why analysis; Pareto

	data. Separate the vital few causes from the trivial many. Confirm causation with data.	triage (42%); antibiotic order requires attending sign-off (31%); pharmacy turnaround >45 min (27%)	chart; scatter plot; hypothesis testing; process capability analysis
I Improve	Design and test solutions that address root causes. Pilot before full implementation. Validate improvement with data.	Solutions: AI-powered sepsis screening at triage; nurse-initiated antibiotic protocol; pharmacy STAT sepsis pathway. Pilot shows 78% cases < 60 min.	Design of Experiments (DOE); FMEA; pilot planning; solution selection matrix; implementation planning; change management
C Control	Implement controls to sustain the improvement. Monitor performance. Hand off to process owner with documented standard.	Control plan: AI alert monitors compliance; monthly dashboard review; nursing competency check; standard operating procedure documented and trained	Control chart (SPC); control plan document; standard operating procedure; training plan; response plan for out-of-control signals

9.5 Case Examples: Lean Six Sigma in Hospitals

Abstract methodology becomes concrete through examples. The following cases: drawn from real hospital improvement work in both US and Indian contexts, demonstrate the kind of results that Lean Six Sigma delivers when applied with discipline and leadership commitment.

Case 1	ED WAIT TIME REDUCTION, US Community Hospital: A 250-bed community hospital in the US Midwest applied Lean Value Stream Mapping to its ED patient journey. The current-state map revealed 14 distinct waiting points averaging 4.2 hours total ED time. The improvement team redesigned triage, implemented a split-flow model for lower-acuity patients, co-located a fast-track area, and implemented AI-powered bed management. Results: median ED time reduced from 4.2 hours to 1.8 hours. Left-without-being-seen

	rate dropped from 8.2% to 1.1%. Patient satisfaction scores improved from 67th to 91st percentile nationally. Sustained over 3 years.
Case 2	OT UTILIZATION IMPROVEMENT, Indian Tertiary Care Hospital: A 600-bed hospital in Maharashtra applied Six Sigma DMAIC to operating theatre underutilization. Baseline: 58% OT utilization with first-case-of-day start delays averaging 47 minutes. Root cause analysis identified: patient preparation delays (38%), surgeon late arrival (29%), equipment unavailability (21%), anesthesia delays (12%). Solutions: standardized pre-operative checklist, mandatory briefing 30 minutes pre-case, instrument tracking system. Result: OT utilization increased to 82%, first-case delay reduced to 8 minutes, generating significant additional surgical revenue while reducing overtime costs.
Case 3	MEDICATION ERROR REDUCTION, Multi-Site Health System: A 4-hospital health system applied Lean Six Sigma to medication administration errors. Baseline error rate: 4.7 errors per 1,000 doses administered. DMAIC analysis identified the top three error types: wrong time (41%), wrong dose (33%), wrong patient (26%). Solutions: BCMA implementation system-wide, smart pump drug library standardization, nurse distraction reduction protocol (no-interruption zones during medication administration). Result: error rate reduced to 0.8 per 1,000 doses, an 83% reduction. Sustained at 18-month follow-up. Estimated 340 preventable adverse drug events avoided annually.

9.6 Building a Lean Six Sigma Program: From Initiative to Culture

The difference between a hospital that runs occasional Lean projects and a hospital that has genuinely transformed through Lean Six Sigma is culture. Projects end. Culture sustains. Building a Lean Six Sigma culture in a healthcare institution requires sustained, visible leadership commitment, structured training programs, dedicated improvement infrastructure, and measurement systems that track improvement outcomes.

The Lean Six Sigma Healthcare Program: Essential Infrastructure

- Leadership champion: a senior executive (ideally the CEO or CMO) who personally leads improvement initiatives, attends improvement events, and reviews improvement metrics in management meetings
- Trained improvement practitioners: Black Belts (full-time improvement leaders for complex projects), Green Belts (part-time improvement leaders embedded in departments), and Yellow Belts (front-line staff with foundational Lean Six Sigma knowledge)
- Improvement management system: a structured system for project identification, prioritization, tracking, and reporting, ensuring improvement effort is aligned with strategic priorities
- Training program: tiered training from awareness (all staff) through Yellow Belt (department champions) through Green Belt (improvement team leaders) through Black Belt (improvement program leaders)
- Visual management: improvement boards in every department showing current performance, improvement goals, and active projects, making quality visible to everyone
- Recognition and celebration: explicit recognition of improvement teams and their results, embedding the message that improvement is valued, seen, and rewarded

★ KEY TAKEAWAYS

8. Lean Six Sigma combines waste elimination (Lean) with variance reduction (Six Sigma): both are necessary for world-class healthcare quality.
9. The eight wastes, TIMWOODS, provide a systematic lens for identifying improvement opportunities in any clinical or operational process.
10. Core Lean tools, Value Stream Mapping, 5S, and Kaizen, produce rapid, visible improvements that build the improvement culture.
11. DMAIC is the disciplined problem-solving framework that ensures solutions address root causes, not symptoms, with data-driven rigor.
12. Real hospital case examples demonstrate consistent results: 50-80% reductions in wait times, errors, and waste when Lean Six Sigma is applied with commitment.
13. The goal is culture, not projects: a trained workforce that continuously improves every process, every day, not occasional consultant-driven initiatives.
14. Medical students and all clinical staff must be trained in Lean Six Sigma: improvement is a professional competency, not a management specialty.

▶ COMING NEXT

Chapter 10 completes Part 3 by bringing together quality management and artificial intelligence into an integrated system, showing how AI enhances quality measurement, how Lean Six Sigma principles govern AI implementation, and how to build the quality-driven AI hospital that can sustain world-class performance.

Chapter 10

Building a Quality-Driven AI System

How Quality Management Principles Govern AI, and How AI Supercharges Quality, in the World-Class Hospital

> *"Improvement usually means doing something that we have never done before."*
>
> **Shigeo Shingo, Toyota production system pioneer. In healthcare, AI enables us to improve in ways that were never previously possible.**

10.1 Introduction: Two Disciplines That Need Each Other

Artificial intelligence and quality management are not competing approaches to hospital improvement. They are complementary disciplines that together create capabilities neither can achieve alone. Quality management without AI is limited by human capacity: the number of data points a quality team can analyze, the speed at which problems can be detected, and the scale at which improvement can be monitored. AI without quality management is dangerous because algorithms deployed without structured governance, validated processes, and continuous monitoring become liabilities rather than assets.

This chapter shows healthcare leaders how to build the integration by creating a quality-driven AI system in which quality management principles govern every aspect of AI deployment, and AI capabilities enhance every dimension of quality measurement and improvement. This is the operating model of the truly world-class hospital: one where human judgment, disciplined quality processes, and intelligent technology work together in a unified system of continuous improvement.

10.2 Quality Management as the Governance Framework for AI

Every AI system deployed in a healthcare organization is, by definition, a process. It has inputs (data), a transformation (the algorithm), and outputs (recommendations, alerts, predictions). And like every clinical process, it must be designed, standardized, measured, monitored, and continuously improved. The quality management principles that govern clinical processes apply with equal force to AI systems.

This is not merely a theoretical proposition. Healthcare AI systems have failed, sometimes catastrophically, when deployed without quality governance. The Epic Sepsis Model, deployed at hundreds of hospitals across the United States, was found in a study published in JAMA Internal Medicine to have substantially lower real-world performance than its validation metrics suggested, in part because the model was not continuously monitored for performance drift, and in part because its alert design contributed to alert fatigue that undermined its clinical impact. The lesson is not that AI is unreliable. The lesson is that AI requires the same structured governance as any clinical process.

The PDCA Cycle Applied to AI Systems

The Plan-Do-Check-Act (PDCA) cycle, the foundational tool of continuous improvement in quality management, provides the governance structure for AI system management:

	Phase	Applied to AI Deployment
P Plan	Select AI system, validate performance, define KPIs, design clinical workflow integration, train staff, and establish governance	Needs assessment; vendor evaluation; local validation study; clinical champion identification; training program design; ethics review
D Do	Pilot the AI system in a defined department or patient population; implement with full monitoring and staff support	Phased deployment; super-user identification; help desk support; daily check-ins with clinical team; incident reporting for AI-related concerns
C Check	Measure AI performance against defined KPIs; compare to pre-implementation baseline; assess clinical adoption and alert response rates	Monthly performance dashboard review; sensitivity/specificity monitoring; clinician override rate analysis; patient outcome tracking; bias auditing
A Act	Based on performance data: optimize alert thresholds, retrain model on local data, expand to additional departments, or escalate concerns	Threshold recalibration; model retraining with new data; workflow redesign; governance committee review; escalation protocol for underperforming systems

10.3 Standardization and Automation: The AI-Quality Intersection

Standardization is the cornerstone of quality management. A process that is performed differently by different people at different times cannot be measured, cannot be reliably improved, and cannot be safely automated. Standardization is the prerequisite for automation, and AI is the most powerful automation tool ever applied to healthcare.

This creates a critical sequence that every healthcare leader must understand: standardize first, then automate. An AI system built on top of a non-standardized process will automate the chaos, producing unreliable results at scale and faster than any human error could. The hospital that attempts to deploy AI in a clinical area where processes are poorly defined, inconsistently followed, and inadequately measured will find that AI amplifies its problems rather than solving them.

The correct sequence is: map the current process → identify and eliminate waste (Lean) → reduce variance and define the standard (Six Sigma) → document the standard as a protocol → implement the protocol with training → measure compliance and outcomes → then deploy AI to automate compliance monitoring, detect deviations, and optimize the standardized process further.

The Standardize-Then-Automate Sequence, Applied Examples

- Sepsis: Standardize the Hour-1 Bundle protocol → achieve consistent manual compliance → deploy AI sepsis prediction alert → monitor AI-triggered bundle initiation rate → use AI data to further optimize the bundle
- Medication administration: Standardize the five rights check → eliminate variation in medication preparation procedures → implement BCMA automation → use AI to analyze dispensing patterns and predict high-risk administration events
- Surgical scheduling: Standardize surgical case scheduling criteria → eliminate ad-hoc scheduling decisions → implement AI scheduling optimization → use AI-generated scheduling data to continuously refine block time allocation
- Radiology reporting: Standardize report structure and turnaround time expectations → reduce variation in reporting practice → implement AI-assisted preliminary reads → use AI data to monitor radiologist performance variation and identify training needs
- Discharge planning: Standardize discharge criteria and planning process → implement structured discharge checklist → deploy AI readmission prediction on admission → use AI risk scores to prioritize discharge planning resources to highest-risk patients

10.4 Measurement and KPIs: AI Enhancing Quality Intelligence

Quality measurement in the traditional model is labor-intensive: quality coordinators manually review charts, extract data from multiple systems, compile reports, and present findings weeks or months after the events they describe. This latency makes quality data descriptive. It tells leaders what happened, but it does not provide predictive or real-time insight.

AI transforms quality measurement in three fundamental ways. First, it makes measurement continuous and automatic quality indicators can be calculated from EHR data in real time without manual abstraction. Second, it enables measurement at a scale that was previously impossible, every patient, every encounter, every process step, rather than a sample. Third, it shifts measurement from descriptive to predictive, AI can identify which patients are likely to experience a quality failure before it occurs, enabling proactive intervention.

Traditional Measurement	AI-Enhanced Measurement	Implementation Requirements
• Monthly or quarterly data cycles • Manual chart abstraction, slow and sampling-dependent • Descriptive, tells you what happened • Limited to measurable processes • Quality team dependent, scalability constrained	• Real-time and continuous • Automated extraction from EHR, complete population coverage • Predictive, identifies risk before events occur • Extends to complex clinical patterns • Scalable to any volume of patients and processes	• High-quality, complete EHR data • Validated AI algorithms with local calibration • Defined quality KPI framework • Clinical governance committee • Dashboard and alert infrastructure • Training for quality teams and clinicians • Continuous monitoring and

• Reactive, review after the fact • Single-institution perspective	• Proactive, enables pre-event intervention • Multi-site benchmarking and learning	improvement process

10.5 Management Reviews: The Governance Cadence

Quality data, however sophisticated the AI system generating it, has no value unless it is reviewed by the people who have the authority and accountability to act on it. The management review cadence is the governance structure that converts data into decisions and decisions into action.

A world-class hospital quality governance structure operates at four levels, each with defined frequency, scope, and accountability:

Daily	Safety huddles at unit level (15 minutes): yesterday's safety events, current high-risk patients, staffing concerns, AI alerts requiring clinical review. Attended by charge nurse and unit leadership. Action items resolved the same day or escalated to a weekly review.
Weekly	Department quality review (30-60 minutes): AI quality dashboard review, trend analysis for key indicators, active incident reviews, and Lean improvement project status. Attended by the department head, quality coordinator, and medical lead. Action items tracked with owner and deadline.
Monthly	Hospital quality committee (2 hours): all department quality reports, adverse event reviews with root cause analysis, quality KPI performance vs. targets, improvement project results, and AI system performance reports. Attended by CMO, CNO, department heads, and quality director. Results shared with board quality committee.

Quarterly	Board quality committee and full management review: strategic quality performance review, accreditation readiness, benchmarking against national/international peers, AI governance review, including bias auditing, major improvement initiative results, capital investment recommendations for quality infrastructure.

10.6 The Quality-AI Integration Matrix, A Practical Framework

The following matrix shows healthcare leaders how quality management systems and AI applications integrate across every major dimension of hospital operations. This is the blueprint for the quality-driven AI hospital.

System / Layer	Quality Management Role	AI Integration Point
Clinical Quality Systems	Evidence-based order sets; clinical pathways; care bundles; protocol adherence monitoring	AI recommends protocol adherence in real time, detects deviations, and predicts outcome risk when protocols are not followed
Patient Safety Systems	Incident reporting; root cause analysis; near-miss tracking; safety huddles; safety culture surveys	AI identifies high-risk patients before incidents occur; analyzes incident patterns for system-level learning; monitors safety indicator trends continuously
Performance Measurement	KPI dashboard; balanced scorecard; benchmarking; accreditation metrics; regulatory reporting	AI automates indicator calculation; enables real-time dashboards; provides predictive performance forecasting; supports automated regulatory reporting
Lean Improvement Programs	Value stream mapping; Kaizen events; 5S; standard work; visual management; improvement boards	AI identifies waste patterns across large datasets impossible to see manually; measures improvement impact in real time; sustains standard work through automated compliance monitoring
Six Sigma Projects	DMAIC methodology; statistical process control; root cause analysis; measurement system analysis	AI provides continuous SPC monitoring for all critical processes; identifies assignable causes in real time; accelerates the

		Analyze phase with pattern recognition across millions of data points
Workforce Quality Development	Competency assessment; training completion tracking; performance management; peer review	AI personalizes training recommendations based on individual performance gaps; monitors skill application in clinical practice; identifies coaching opportunities
Supply Chain Quality	Vendor qualification, product quality monitoring; inventory management; recall management	AI-powered demand forecasting; automated vendor performance scoring; predictive maintenance for medical equipment; real-time recall alert management
Patient Experience Management	Patient satisfaction surveys, complaint management; patient advisory councils, and communication training	AI sentiment analysis of patient feedback; real-time patient experience monitoring; automated follow-up for dissatisfied patients; personalized communication optimization

10.7 AI Governance as a Quality Function

One of the most important and most frequently neglected aspects of AI deployment in healthcare is governance, the formal oversight structures that ensure AI systems continue to perform as intended, remain ethically sound, and are managed with the same accountability as any other clinical process.

AI governance must be treated as a quality management function, not merely an IT function or a compliance exercise. It requires clinical leadership, defined processes, continuous measurement, and a culture of transparency about AI performance and limitations.

The AI Governance Framework, Eight Essential Components

- AI governance committee: cross-functional committee with clinical, technical, legal, ethical, and patient representation, reviews all AI deployments and monitors ongoing performance
- Pre-deployment validation: every AI system must be validated on local patient population data before clinical deployment, vendor performance claims are not sufficient
- Performance monitoring: defined KPIs for every AI system (sensitivity, specificity, positive predictive value, alert fatigue rate, clinician override rate) tracked monthly
- Bias auditing: quarterly audit of AI performance across patient demographic groups, gender, age, race/ethnicity, socioeconomic status, to detect and correct disparate performance
- Drift monitoring: AI model performance degrades over time as patient populations and clinical practices change, formal drift detection and retraining protocols are mandatory
- Incident management: defined process for reporting, investigating, and responding to AI-related adverse events or near-misses, with the same rigor as clinical incident management
- Transparency and explainability: clinicians must be able to understand why an AI system generated a specific alert or recommendation, Black-box AI systems without explain ability are not acceptable in clinical settings. Annual review and recertification: every AI system undergoes a formal annual review of performance, clinical utility, patient safety record, and continued appropriateness for deployment

★ KEY TAKEAWAYS

15. AI and quality management are complementary disciplines, AI without quality governance is dangerous, quality management without AI is limited. Together they are transformative.
16. Quality management principles, PDCA, standardization, measurement, continuous improvement, govern AI deployment with the same rigor as any clinical process.
17. The non-negotiable sequence: standardize first, then automate. AI built on non-standardized processes amplifies chaos rather than solving it.
18. AI transforms quality measurement from retrospective and sampled to real-time, comprehensive, and predictive, enabling proactive quality management at scale.
19. The management review cadence, whether daily, weekly, monthly, or quarterly, converts quality data into decisions and decisions into improvement actions.
20. AI governance is a quality function requiring clinical ownership, defined KPIs, bias auditing, drift monitoring, and formal annual recertification.
21. The quality-driven AI hospital integrates quality management and AI across all eight major operational domains: from clinical quality to patient experience to supply chain.
22. The Bhagyoday model demonstrates that this integration is achievable: AI enhances the performance that quality management has already made good, world-class care in practice.

▶ COMING NEXT

Part 4 moves into the regulatory and governance landscape, the rules, standards, and frameworks that govern both healthcare quality and AI use in the United States and India. Understanding these frameworks is essential for every leader building a compliant, safe, and accountable AI-integrated healthcare system.

PART FOUR

Regulations, Standards & Governance

The legal, ethical, and institutional frameworks every healthcare leader must know, for USA and India

Chapter 11

Healthcare Regulations: USA

HIPAA, FDA, Joint Commission, and CMS, What Every Leader Must Know and Do

> *"Compliance is not the ceiling. It is the floor. World-class healthcare organizations exceed every regulatory requirement, because they understand that the purpose of regulation is patient protection, not paperwork."*
>
> **Jay P. Patel Quality & Productivity Solutions, Inc.**

11.1 Introduction: Why Regulation Is a Leadership Responsibility

Healthcare regulation in the United States is one of the most complex regulatory environments in the world. Dozens of federal and state agencies, multiple accreditation bodies, hundreds of specific standards, and an ever-evolving landscape of AI-specific guidance create a compliance burden that can feel overwhelming, particularly for leaders trying to simultaneously manage clinical operations, drive quality improvement, and implement new technologies.

The temptation is to delegate regulatory compliance to a compliance officer and move on. This is a mistake. In healthcare, regulatory compliance is not a legal department function. It is a leadership function, because the regulations exist to protect patients, and patient protection is the core responsibility of every healthcare leader. Understanding the major US regulatory frameworks, what they require, why they exist, and how they interact with AI and with one another, is essential knowledge for every executive, medical director, and department leader.

This chapter provides that knowledge: clear, practical, and organized around what leaders need to know and do, not what lawyers need to defend in court.

11.2 HIPAA: Protecting Patient Privacy in the Digital and AI Era

The Health Insurance Portability and Accountability Act (HIPAA), enacted in 1996 and significantly strengthened by the HITECH Act of 2009 and the Omnibus Rule of 2013, is the foundational federal law governing the privacy and security of patient health information in the United States. Every healthcare provider, health plan, healthcare clearinghouse, and their business associates, including AI vendors, must comply with HIPAA.

HIPAA, At a Glance
Full Name: Health Insurance Portability and Accountability Act (1996), enhanced by HITECH (2009) and Omnibus Rule (2013)
Enforced By: HHS Office for Civil Rights (OCR), investigates complaints and conducts audits
Who Must Comply: Covered entities (providers, health plans, clearinghouses) and all business associates (including AI vendors, cloud providers, EHR vendors)
Core Requirement: Protect the privacy and security of Protected Health Information (PHI), any individually identifiable health information
Key Rules: Privacy Rule (use and disclosure of PHI); Security Rule (administrative, physical, and technical safeguards for electronic PHI); Breach Notification Rule (notification within 60 days of breach)
Penalties: Civil: $100 to $50,000 per violation, up to $1.9 million per violation category per year. Criminal: up to $250,000 and 10 years imprisonment for willful violations
AI Implication: Every AI system that accesses, processes, or generates PHI is subject to HIPAA. Business Associate Agreements (BAAs) required with all AI vendors

HIPAA and AI: The Critical Requirements

The deployment of AI in healthcare creates new and complex HIPAA compliance considerations that every leader must understand:

- Business Associate Agreements: Every AI vendor that has access to PHI, whether for model training, system operation, or quality monitoring, must sign a HIPAA-compliant Business Associate Agreement (BAA). This is non-negotiable. Without a BAA, there should be no PHI access. De-identification for model training: If patient data is used to train AI models, it must either be fully de-identified according to HIPAA's Safe Harbor or Expert Determination standards, or covered by a valid authorization or waiver. Using identifiable PHI to train AI without a proper legal basis is a HIPAA violation.
- Minimum necessary standard: AI systems should be configured to access only the minimum amount of PHI necessary for their intended function. A scheduling AI does not need access to psychiatric records. A radiology AI does not need access to financial information.
- Security safeguards for AI systems: AI systems that process ePHI must implement the full HIPAA Security Rule requirements, access controls, audit logs, encryption, integrity controls, and transmission security. These requirements apply to AI systems with the same force as EHR systems.
- Patient rights in the AI context: Patients retain all HIPAA rights, including the right to access their records, regardless of whether AI systems are involved in their care. If an AI system generates a clinical document or recommendation, patients can request that record. If an AI is used in a decision affecting their care, patients can request a human review.

HIPAA Compliance Action Plan for AI-Implementing Hospitals

- Conduct a HIPAA Risk Analysis specific to every AI system before deployment, document identified risks and mitigations
- Require executed BAAs from every AI vendor, cloud provider, and technology partner with PHI access before the system goes live

- Establish a PHI inventory that includes all AI systems, databases, and data flows, updated whenever new AI systems are deployed
- Implement role-based access controls for all AI systems, clinical AI accessible only to authorized clinical staff
- Configure audit logging for all AI system access to PHI, logs must be reviewed regularly and retained per HIPAA requirements
- Train all staff annually on HIPAA, with specific modules on AI-related privacy obligations updated as AI deployments evolve
- Establish and test a Breach Response Plan, with specific protocols for AI-related breaches (e.g., model inversion attacks, unauthorized data access through AI interfaces)

11.3 FDA Regulation of AI and Medical Devices

The US Food and Drug Administration (FDA) regulates medical devices, and increasingly, AI and machine learning-based software used in clinical decision-making is classified as a medical device subject to FDA oversight. This is one of the most rapidly evolving areas of healthcare regulation, and one of the most important for leaders implementing clinical AI.

FDA AI/ML Regulation, At a Glance
Regulatory Framework: Medical Device Amendments; 21st Century Cures Act; FDA Software as a Medical Device (SaMD) guidance; AI/ML Action Plan (2021)
Key Classification: Software as a Medical Device (SaMD): software intended to diagnose, treat, prevent, or monitor a disease or condition. This includes many AI clinical decision support tools
Risk-Based Approach: Class I (low risk, general controls), Class II (moderate risk, 510(k) clearance), Class III (high risk, PMA approval), AI tools classified based on intended use and risk to patients

510(k) Clearance: Most AI diagnostic tools cleared via 510(k), demonstrating substantial equivalence to a predicate device already on the market
De Novo Pathway: Novel AI devices without predicates may use De Novo classification, establishing new regulatory classification for first-of-kind AI tools
Predetermined Change Control Plan: Proposed framework allowing AI/ML-based SaMD to change and improve over time within FDA-approved parameters, addressing AI's inherent adaptability
Post-Market Monitoring: FDA increasingly requires real-world performance monitoring for cleared AI devices, manufacturers must report adverse events and performance data

What Healthcare Leaders Must Know About FDA and AI

For hospital leaders implementing AI, FDA regulation has three practical implications:

- Verify FDA status before deployment: Any AI tool used for clinical decision-making, diagnosis, treatment recommendations, patient monitoring, should be evaluated for FDA clearance status. Deploying non-cleared AI in clinical decision roles creates regulatory, liability, and patient safety risks.
- Clinical decision support vs. locked-down tools: The FDA distinguishes between non-device clinical decision support (software that simply displays information for clinician interpretation) and SaMD (software that drives or informs clinical decisions). Many AI vendors claim their tools are non-device CDS to avoid FDA oversight, leaders should understand this distinction and evaluate claims critically.
- Post-market vigilance: Even FDA-cleared AI devices require post-market surveillance. Leaders must establish processes for monitoring AI performance in their specific patient population, reporting adverse events to the FDA, and updating AI systems when performance issues are identified.

11.4 The Joint Commission: Standards for Quality and Patient Safety

The Joint Commission (TJC) is the largest and most widely recognized hospital accreditation organization in the United States, accrediting more than 22,000 healthcare organizations. Joint Commission accreditation is recognized by CMS as meeting Medicare/Medicaid Conditions of Participation, making it both a quality and a financial necessity for most US hospitals. The Joint Commission's standards directly intersect with AI implementation in several critical areas.

National Patient Safety Goals	Leadership & Governance Standards	Information Management Standards
• NPSG 01.01.01: Identify patients correctly, AI patient identification tools must meet this standard • NPSG 02.03.01: Report critical results of tests, AI result delivery systems must meet timing requirements • NPSG 03.04.01: Label medications accurately, AI medication systems must support this standard • NPSG 06.01.01: Improve alarm safety, AI-generated	• LD.03.06.01: Leaders create and maintain a culture of safety and quality, includes AI governance • LD.04.01.01: Operational planning addresses patient safety and quality, AI strategy must be included • Leaders are accountable for compliance of all technology systems used in patient care • Vendor oversight: Joint Commission expects leaders to evaluate and	• IM.02.02.01: Information confidentiality, security, and integrity, applies to AI systems handling patient data • IM.01.01.03: Planning for the management of information, AI data flows must be included in IM planning • Downtime procedures required, AI system downtime must have defined clinical workarounds • Information management training, staff

clinical alerts subject to alarm management standards • NPSG 15.01.01: Suicide risk reduction, AI screening tools must meet clinical validation requirements	monitor technology vendors • AI systems must be part of the hospital's formal risk management program	must be trained on all information systems including AI • Audit trails: Joint Commission expects evidence of controlled information access including AI system access logs

11.5 CMS: Value-Based Care and Quality Reporting

The Centers for Medicare and Medicaid Services (CMS) is the largest payer in the US healthcare system, covering approximately 160 million Americans through Medicare, Medicaid, and CHIP. CMS quality programs directly affect hospital revenue and create strong financial incentives for quality improvement that increasingly align with AI capabilities.

Key CMS Quality Programs: Financial Impact for Hospitals

- Hospital Value-Based Purchasing (VBP): adjusts Medicare payments (+/- up to 2%) based on performance on quality, safety, efficiency, and patient experience measures, AI-enhanced performance directly improves VBP scores
- Hospital Readmissions Reduction Program (HRRP): penalties of up to 3% of all Medicare payments for excess readmissions, AI readmission prediction and prevention programs directly reduce this penalty exposure
- Hospital-Acquired Condition (HAC) Reduction Program: 1% payment penalty for hospitals in the worst quartile for HAC rates, AI early warning for HAIs, falls, and pressure injuries reduces HAC rates

- Merit-Based Incentive Payment System (MIPS): for physician practices, AI-assisted documentation, quality reporting, and care coordination improve MIPS performance scores
- Promoting Interoperability: CMS program rewarding hospitals for EHR meaningful use and FHIR-based data sharing, directly incentivizes the digital infrastructure that AI requires
- Quality Payment Program: value-based payment models (ACOs, bundled payments) reward coordinated, high-quality care, AI population health management supports performance in these models

11.6 Real-World Reflection: Regulatory Readiness as Competitive Advantage

Healthcare leaders who view regulatory compliance as a burden to be minimized are missing a fundamental strategic insight: regulatory readiness is a competitive advantage. Hospitals that achieve and exceed Joint Commission standards, maintain strong CMS quality scores, implement HIPAA-compliant AI, and stay ahead of FDA guidance on medical AI are not just compliant; they are demonstrably better hospitals.

They have lower readmission rates, fewer adverse events, better patient experience scores, and stronger financial performance, all of which are simultaneously the outcomes of good quality management, the requirements of regulatory standards, and the results that AI can help achieve when properly implemented.

The regulatory framework for healthcare in the United States, complex as it is, points in exactly the right direction: toward safer, more effective, more patient-centered, more equitable care. The leader's job is not to fight that direction but to navigate it skillfully, using quality management tools, AI capabilities, and skilled leadership to build organizations that achieve regulatory requirements as a byproduct of genuine excellence.

★ KEY TAKEAWAYS

1. HIPAA is the foundational patient privacy law, every AI system accessing PHI requires BAAs, risk analysis, security safeguards, and staff training.
2. FDA increasingly regulates clinical AI as Software as a Medical Device (SaMD), leaders must verify FDA clearance status before deploying clinical decision-making AI.
3. The Joint Commission's standards for patient safety, leadership, and information management all apply directly to AI systems, compliance requires active AI governance.
4. CMS quality programs (VBP, HRRP, HAC) create direct financial incentives for the quality improvements that AI delivers, understanding these linkages builds the business case for AI investment.
5. Regulatory compliance is not the ceiling; it is the floor. World-class hospitals exceed regulatory requirements as a natural result of genuine quality excellence.
6. Regulatory readiness is a competitive advantage: HIPAA-compliant, FDA-cleared, Joint Commission-accredited, CMS high-performing hospitals are measurably better, and financially stronger.

▶ COMING NEXT

Chapter 12 turns to India, examining the NABH accreditation system, the National Digital Health Mission, CDSCO medical device regulations, and the Ayushman Bharat program that is transforming healthcare access for 500 million Indians.

Chapter 12

Healthcare Regulations: India

NABH, National Digital Health Mission, CDSCO, and Ayushman Bharat, Building World-Class Care at National Scale

> *"India has the potential to leapfrog decades of healthcare infrastructure development, if its leaders make the right choices now about digital systems, quality standards, and equitable access."*
>
> **Jay P. Patel on the unique opportunity that India's healthcare transformation represents for the world.**

12.1 Introduction: India's Regulatory Landscape: Complex, Evolving, and Critical

India's healthcare regulatory environment is among the most ambitious and complex in the world. A country of 1.4 billion people, with extraordinary diversity in geography, language, income, and healthcare infrastructure, is attempting to build a unified, high-quality, digitally integrated healthcare system through a combination of accreditation standards, national digital health programs, medical device regulation, and universal health coverage initiatives.

The pace of regulatory evolution in India is remarkable. In just the past decade, the country has launched the National Digital Health Mission, enacted the Digital Personal Data Protection Act, expanded the Ayushman Bharat health insurance program to cover 500 million people, and developed new guidance for AI and medical devices through CDSCO. For healthcare leaders in India, and for global leaders working with Indian institutions understanding this regulatory landscape is essential. It forms the foundation for building institutions that are both compliant and world-class. This chapter examines the four most important regulatory and programmatic frameworks for Indian healthcare: NABH accreditation, the

National Digital Health Mission, CDSCO medical device and AI regulation, and the Ayushman Bharat program.

12.2 NABH: The Quality Accreditation Standard for Indian Hospitals

The National Accreditation Board for Hospitals and Healthcare Providers (NABH) is the premier hospital accreditation body in India, operating under the Quality Council of India (QCI). NABH accreditation is recognized by insurance companies, government health programs, and international health tourism patients as evidence that a hospital meets defined quality and safety standards.

NABH, At a Glance
Established: 2006 under the Quality Council of India, now accredits over 900 hospitals across India
International Recognition: Member of the International Society for Quality in Health Care (ISQua), NABH standards internationally benchmarked
Standards Structure: 11 chapters covering Patient-Centered Standards and Organization-Centered Standards, 100 standards, 636 measurable elements
Entry Level Programme: Progressive pathway, Entry Level (small hospitals), Accreditation (full standards), Advanced (highest level of compliance)
Survey Process: Application, pre-assessment, document review, on-site survey by trained assessors, decision by NABH board
Benefits: Insurance empanelment eligibility, government scheme participation, patient trust, staff professional development, systematic quality improvement
AI Implication: NABH increasingly incorporates digital health requirements, EHR standards, patient data privacy, information security now explicit in accreditation criteria

NABH Standards Most Relevant to AI and Digital Implementation

NABH's 11 standard chapters contain requirements that directly govern how AI and digital systems must be managed in accredited hospitals:

NABH Standard Chapter	AI and Digital Health Requirements
Access, Assessment and Continuity of Care (AAC)	Clinical decision support tools must be validated; triage processes must be standardized; AI-assisted assessment tools must meet clinical evidence requirements
Care of Patients (COP)	Evidence-based care protocols required; AI-assisted protocol monitoring must support compliance tracking; clinical pathway adherence measurable
Management of Medication (MOM)	Medication management system must prevent errors; AI medication interaction checking and barcode administration verification meet MOM standards
Patient Rights and Education (PRE)	Patients must be informed about their care; AI use in clinical decisions should be disclosed; informed consent processes must be documented
Hospital Infection Control (HIC)	AI infection surveillance tools must support the HAI monitoring required by HIC standards; automated outbreak detection directly addresses HIC requirements
Continuous Quality Improvement (CQI)	Quality improvement program required, AI-powered quality measurement and Lean Six Sigma programs directly meet CQI requirements

Responsibilities of Management (ROM)	Leadership must demonstrate active quality oversight, AI governance committee and quality dashboard reviews meet ROM leadership requirements
Information Management System (IMS)	EHR and information systems must be secure, accessible, and accurate; HIPAA-equivalent patient data privacy is required; AI system data governance addresses IMS standards

12.3 National Digital Health Mission (NDHM): India's Digital Health Architecture

The National Digital Health Mission (NDHM), launched in 2020 and now operating under the Ayushman Bharat Digital Mission (ABDM), is India's ambitious initiative to create a unified digital health ecosystem across the country. Its goal is to ensure that every Indian has a unique Health ID, that health records are portable and accessible across providers, and that digital health infrastructure supports the delivery of high-quality care to every citizen.

National Digital Health Mission / ABDM, At a Glance
Launched: August 2020 (pilot); national rollout 2021, governed by the Ministry of Health and Family Welfare
Ayushman Bharat Health Account (ABHA): Unique 14-digit Health ID for every Indian, enables portable, longitudinal health records linked across providers
Healthcare Professionals Registry (HPR): National registry of all licensed healthcare professionals, enables credential verification and patient-provider linkage
Health Facility Registry (HFR): National registry of all health facilities, public and private, with standardized identifiers for care coordination

Unified Health Interface (UHI): Open network for digital health services, telehealth, appointment booking, prescription sharing across providers and platforms
Technical Standards: HL7 FHIR R4 adopted as the national health data exchange standard; SNOMED CT for clinical terminology; DICOM for imaging
Data Privacy Framework: Governed by the Digital Personal Data Protection Act 2023 (DPDPA), India's comprehensive personal data protection law
AI Opportunity: ABDM creates the national data infrastructure that AI population health tools require: unified, standardized, longitudinal patient data at a national scale

What ABDM Means for Hospital Leaders in India

For hospital leaders in India, ABDM participation is no longer optional; it is increasingly a requirement for government scheme empanelment and is becoming a prerequisite for NABH accreditation at higher levels. More importantly, ABDM participation is the path to the digital infrastructure that AI requires.

- Register all facilities in the Health Facility Registry (HFR); this is the first step to ABDM participation and is straightforward for most institutions
- Implement ABHA ID creation at registration, enable patients to create or link their Health ID at every encounter, building the portable record infrastructure
- Adopt FHIR-compliant EHR systems, ABDM-compliant EHR is the technical foundation for data sharing, AI integration, and accreditation compliance
- Train all clinical staff on ABDM, patients will increasingly arrive with ABHA IDs and expect digital health records to follow them; staff must understand how to access and contribute to these records
- Engage with the Unified Health Interface, position your institution to offer telemedicine and digital services through the UHI, extending your reach to patients across geographies

12.4 CDSCO: Regulating AI Medical Devices in India

The Central Drugs Standard Control Organisation (CDSCO), India's equivalent to the US FDA, is responsible for regulating medical devices, including AI-powered software used in clinical settings. India's medical device regulatory framework has been rapidly evolving: the Medical Devices Rules 2017 brought AI software within the regulatory scope, and CDSCO has been developing specific guidance for AI/ML-based medical devices in collaboration with international regulatory bodies.

FDA (USA), AI Device Regulation	CDSCO (India), AI Device Regulation
Established framework with decades of precedent for software/medical device regulation	Evolving framework, Medical Devices Rules 2017 is foundation; AI-specific guidance under development
510(k) clearance for moderate-risk AI; PMA for high-risk; De Novo for novel devices	Class A (low risk), Class B (moderate), Class C (moderate-high), Class D (high risk), most AI devices Class B/C
Predetermined Change Control Plan allows AI adaptation within approved parameters	Guidance on AI adaptability still developing, currently requires approval of significant modifications
Post-market surveillance requirements well-defined with mandatory reporting timelines	Post-market requirements developing, adverse event reporting system for devices being strengthened
FDA Digital Health Center of Excellence provides dedicated AI/ML guidance and support	CDSCO developing AI-specific guidance, international collaboration with FDA and other regulators
Key action: verify 510(k) clearance or FDA exemption status for every clinical AI tool	Key action: verify CDSCO registration for medical device AI tools; monitor evolving guidance actively

12.5 Ayushman Bharat: Universal Health Coverage and Quality Implications

Ayushman Bharat is the Indian government's flagship universal health coverage program, operating through two components: Pradhan Mantri Jan Arogya Yojana (PM-JAY), which provides health insurance coverage of up to Rs. 5 lacs per family per year to approximately 500 million people (the bottom 40% of India's population), and Health and Wellness Centres (HWCs) / Ayushman Arogya Mandirs, which are transforming 150,000 sub-health centres and primary health centres into comprehensive primary care facilities.

Ayushman Bharat, Implications for Hospital Quality and AI

- Empanelment requirements: hospitals seeking PM-JAY empanelment must meet defined quality standards, NABH accreditation is a pathway to higher package rates and preferred empanelment status
- Quality-linked payments: PM-JAY package rates are increasingly quality-linked, hospitals with better outcomes and accreditation receive better reimbursement, creating a direct financial incentive for quality investment
- AI opportunity in HWCs: Ayushman Arogya Mandirs are equipped with telemedicine, basic diagnostics, and EHR systems, AI triage, chronic disease management, and remote specialist consultation directly support HWC service delivery
- Population health scale: PM-JAY's 500 million beneficiaries represent the largest population health data opportunity in the world, AI population health tools applied to this data can transform preventive care at a scale unmatched anywhere
- Training requirement: empanelled hospitals must maintain trained clinical staff for all procedures, Lean Six Sigma and AI literacy training programs directly address PM-JAY staffing quality requirements
- Claims management: AI-powered claims processing, fraud detection, and quality auditing are priorities for PM-JAY administrators, hospitals with strong AI-enabled documentation have fewer claim denials and faster payment

12.6 Medical College Accreditation in India: NMC and Beyond

India's regulatory framework does not stop at hospital accreditation. For institutions like Bhagyoday that are both hospitals and medical colleges, a second and equally demanding accreditation framework applies: medical education regulation. The National Medical Commission (NMC), established in 2020 to replace the Medical Council of India, is the apex regulatory body governing medical education across India, and its standards define what a world-class Indian medical college must provide.

Understanding NMC standards is essential for any institution building the next generation of doctors, because the standards determine not just what students are taught, but how they are taught, who teaches them, what infrastructure is required, and increasingly, how digital health and AI must be integrated into the curriculum.

National Medical Commission (NMC), Medical College Standards at a Glance
Established: 2020, replaced the Medical Council of India; governs MBBS, MD/MS, and super-specialty programs across India
Key Regulations: Graduate Medical Education Regulations (GMER); Minimum Standards for Medical Colleges; Competency-Based Medical Education (CBME) curriculum framework
Infrastructure Requirements: Minimum bed strength (150-300 beds, depending on intake); defined faculty: student ratios; clinical labs, simulation centres, library; equipment standards for each specialty
Faculty Standards: Minimum qualifications, experience, and teacher-student ratios defined by NMC; faculty development programs mandatory; visiting faculty limitations
Curriculum Framework: Competency-Based Medical Education (CBME) adopted nationally, outcome-oriented, skill-assessed, attitude-integrated curriculum replacing the knowledge-only approach

AI & Digital Health: NMC's CBME framework increasingly incorporates health informatics, telemedicine, and evidence-based medicine, institutions integrating AI literacy gain competitive edge for future compliance
Assessment: Formative and summative assessment with competency milestones; NEXT (National Exit Test) replacing university exams, standardizing graduate competency nationally
Annual Inspections: Regular inspections by NMC and state medical councils; non-compliant colleges risk intake reduction or derecognition

CBME: The Curriculum Framework That Defines Modern Indian Medical Education

Competency-Based Medical Education (CBME) is NMC's most significant curriculum reform in decades. Adopted in 2019 and now fully implemented across all Indian medical colleges, CBME shifts the focus of medical education from what students are taught to what students can actually do. This shift, from knowledge transmission to competency development, is directly aligned with the world-class medical education philosophy of this book.

CBME defines competencies across three domains: Knowledge (understanding of biomedical and clinical sciences), Skills (clinical, procedural, and communication abilities), and Attitudes and Communication (AETCOM: Attitude, Ethics, and Communication module). The integration of AETCOM as a mandatory curriculum component is particularly significant, it brings the human values dimension into formal medical education requirements, not just as an aspiration but as an assessed competency.

For institutions implementing AI, CBME provides the natural curriculum framework for integrating AI literacy: AI tools can be introduced as part of the clinical skills domain, AI ethics within AETCOM, and health informatics within the community medicine and public health components. The NMC framework does not yet mandate AI education, but institutions that build it in now are preparing their students for the reality of medical practice and positioning themselves ahead of regulatory requirements that are certain to follow.

NMC CBME, Key Competency Areas Relevant to AI and Digital Health Integration

- Health Informatics (FM/Community Medicine): understanding of health information systems, EHR, telemedicine, and digital health tools, the natural home for foundational AI literacy
- Evidence-Based Medicine (across specialties): critical appraisal of evidence, including AI-generated clinical evidence, essential for the AI-critical clinician
- Clinical Decision-Making (Medicine, Surgery, Pediatrics): structured clinical reasoning that must include how to integrate and critically evaluate AI decision support
- Communication Skills (AETCOM): patient communication about AI involvement in care: disclosure, consent, and trust-building in an AI-integrated practice
- Ethics and Professionalism (AETCOM): AI ethics, data privacy, algorithmic accountability, the professional obligations of the AI-era physician
- Quality Improvement (Hospital Administration): Lean, Six Sigma, and quality management tools: directly relevant to AI governance and improvement methodology
- Research Methodology (throughout curriculum): understanding of data, statistics, and study design, foundational for evaluating AI performance claims and published AI research

12.7 Real-World Reflection: Regulatory Compliance as the Foundation at Bhagyoday

At Bhagyoday Hospital and Medical College in Kadi, Gujarat, regulatory compliance is not treated as a constraint on clinical practice; it is treated as the framework that gives clinical practice its credibility and accountability. The institution is pursuing full NABH accreditation with the understanding that NABH represents the minimum standard, not the ultimate aspiration.

ABDM participation is built into the institution's foundational digital architecture, ABHA ID creation is standard practice at registration, FHIR-compliant EHR infrastructure is implemented from inception, and the Health Facility Registry entry was completed as a prerequisite to operations. This early compliance investment means that as ABDM requirements expand, as they inevitably will, Bhagyoday is positioned to meet them with minimal incremental effort.

The institution's engagement with Ayushman Bharat is deliberate and values-driven. Serving PM-JAY beneficiaries, the families in Kadi and the surrounding region who could not otherwise afford quality hospital care, is not just a compliance requirement or a revenue source. It is the expression of the equity value that anchors the institution's mission: world-class care for every patient, regardless of their economic circumstances.

This is what regulatory compliance looks like when it is lived from the inside out, not as a set of rules imposed from outside, but as an expression of values that were always there.

★ KEY TAKEAWAYS

7. NABH accreditation is the quality standard for Indian hospitals, pursue it as the minimum, and build beyond it toward JCI and ISO standards for world-class recognition.
8. ABDM (National Digital Health Mission) creates India's national digital health infrastructure, ABHA ID, FHIR standards, and unified health records are the foundation for AI at a national scale.
9. CDSCO is evolving its AI medical device regulatory framework, leaders must verify device registration status and monitor guidance actively as requirements develop.
10. Ayushman Bharat creates both a quality imperative (empanelment requirements) and an extraordinary AI opportunity (500 million beneficiaries, population health at a national scale).
11. India has a unique opportunity to leapfrog, building AI-ready, NABH-accredited, ABDM-compliant healthcare systems from scratch, avoiding the legacy system burdens that challenge US healthcare.
12. Regulatory compliance lived from the inside, as an expression of values, produces institutions that exceed requirements naturally, because excellence and compliance point in the same direction.

▶ COMING NEXT

Chapter 13 moves to global standards that transcend national boundaries, WHO guidelines, ISO quality standards, and the HL7 FHIR interoperability framework that is becoming the universal language of healthcare data exchange.

Chapter 13

Global Standards in Healthcare

WHO Guidelines, ISO Standards, and HL7 FHIR, The Universal Language of World-Class Care

> *"Health is a state of complete physical, mental, and social well-being and not merely the absence of disease or infirmity."*
>
> **World Health Organization Constitution, 1948. The definition that guides every global health standard.**

13.1 Introduction: Why Global Standards Matter

Healthcare is local in its delivery, every patient encounter happens in a specific place, with specific people, in a specific cultural and institutional context. But the knowledge that drives healthcare is global. The evidence base for clinical practice, the standards for patient safety, the frameworks for quality management, and the technical architectures for digital health do not belong to any single country. They are the collective product of global scientific and professional communities, and every hospital, in every country, benefits from aligning with these global standards rather than reinventing them locally.

For healthcare leaders in the United States and India, global standards serve three practical functions. First, they provide the benchmarks against which to measure performance, what does world-class actually look like, and how do we compare? Second, they provide the frameworks for interoperability, how do our systems communicate with providers, researchers, and public health authorities in other countries? Third, they provide the credibility signals that matter to international patients, medical tourism programs, research collaborations, and global health partnerships.

This chapter examines three bodies of global standards that every healthcare leader must know: WHO guidelines and frameworks, ISO quality and medical device standards, and the HL7 FHIR interoperability standard.

13.2 WHO: Global Health Leadership and Clinical Standards

The World Health Organization (WHO) is the United Nations specialized agency for global public health. Its guidelines, frameworks, and tools set the international baseline for healthcare quality and patient safety. WHO standards are not legally binding, they are adopted voluntarily, but their authority and evidence base make them the reference point for healthcare policy and practice worldwide.

WHO Patient Safety Framework

WHO's Global Patient Safety Action Plan 2021-2030 provides the most comprehensive framework for patient safety that exists at a global scale. Its seven strategic objectives: each with specific actions for health systems, health facilities, and health workers, define what world-class patient safety looks like regardless of national context.

WHO Global Patient Safety Action Plan 2021-2030, Seven Strategic Objectives
• Objective 1, Policies for zero avoidable harm: establish national patient safety policies with clear accountability, resources, and measurement frameworks, includes AI safety governance • Objective 2, High-reliability systems: build health systems that reliably prevent errors through standardization, technology, and safety culture, directly aligned with HRO principles in Chapter 8 • Objective 3, Safety of clinical processes: ensure that every clinical process, from diagnosis to treatment to discharge, is designed to minimize error and maximize safety • Objective 4, Patient and family engagement: involve patients and families as active partners in safety, not passive recipients

of care, through education, transparency, and shared decision-making

- Objective 5, Health worker education and skills: ensure that all health workers have the safety knowledge and skills their roles require, including AI literacy and human factors training
- Objective 6, Information, research, and risk management: build the data infrastructure and analytical capability to understand, learn from, and prevent patient safety failures
- Objective 7, Synergies and innovation: leverage technology, including AI, to advance patient safety goals, with ethical governance ensuring innovation serves patients

WHO Essential Medicines and Clinical Guidelines

WHO's Model Lists of Essential Medicines and its clinical treatment guidelines represent the global evidence base for appropriate, effective, and equitable clinical care. Hospitals in both the United States and India that align their formularies and clinical protocols with WHO guidance ensure that their care meets the highest global evidence standards.

In the context of AI, WHO guidelines serve as the evidence base against which AI clinical decision support should be calibrated. An AI recommendation that diverges from WHO guidelines should be explainable, and if it cannot be explained, it should be reviewed carefully before clinical deployment.

WHO Guidelines on AI for Health

In 2021, the WHO published its landmark guidance: 'Ethics and Governance of Artificial Intelligence for Health.' This document establishes six core principles for ethical AI in healthcare that have been widely adopted by national regulatory bodies, including the FDA and CDSCO, and that should govern AI governance committees in every hospital implementing AI.

WHO AI Principle	What It Means in Practice	Hospital Action Required
• 1. Protecting human autonomy • 2. Promoting human well-being and safety • 3. Ensuring transparency and explainability • 4. Fostering responsibility and accountability • 5. Ensuring inclusiveness and equity • 6. Promoting AI that is responsive and sustainable	• Patients control their data; humans make final clinical decisions • AI safety evaluation before deployment; ongoing monitoring • AI recommendations explainable to clinicians and patients • Clear accountability chain: vendor, hospital, clinician • AI performs equally across patient demographic groups • AI systems should adapt to changing needs without losing reliability	• Establish patient data consent framework; ensure human oversight • Pre-deployment validation; AI adverse event reporting • Select explainable AI; train staff to interrogate AI outputs • Define AI governance roles; board-level AI oversight • Mandatory bias auditing; diverse training data requirements • Annual AI system review; update plan for model maintenance

13.3 ISO Standards: The Global Quality and Safety Framework

The International Organization for Standardization (ISO) develops internationally agreed standards that apply across industries and countries. In healthcare, three ISO standards are particularly important for leaders implementing quality management systems and AI: ISO 9001 (Quality Management Systems), ISO 13485 (Medical Devices Quality Management), and ISO 27001 (Information Security Management).

ISO 9001:2015	Quality Management Systems, the most widely applied management standard in the world, applicable to any organization including healthcare. The seven principles of ISO 9001: customer focus, leadership, engagement of people, process approach, improvement, evidence-based decision making, and relationship management, are the structural equivalent of everything described in Part 3 of this book. ISO 9001 certification demonstrates to patients, payers, and partners that your quality management system is systematically designed, documented, monitored, and continuously improved. In healthcare, ISO 9001 often complements accreditation (NABH/Joint Commission) by providing the underlying quality management system structure that accreditation standards require.
ISO 13485:2016	Medical Devices Quality Management Systems, the specific ISO standard for organizations involved in the design, manufacture, installation, and servicing of medical devices, including AI medical device software. Hospitals that develop AI tools internally, or that modify commercially available AI systems for local use, may need to consider ISO 13485 compliance. More importantly, AI vendors supplying SaMD to hospitals should be ISO 13485 certified; this is a meaningful quality credential that leaders should require during vendor evaluation.
ISO 27001:2022	Information Security Management Systems, the global standard for information security management, directly applicable to healthcare organizations managing patient data

	and AI systems. ISO 27001 certification provides internationally recognized evidence that an organization has implemented a comprehensive, risk-based approach to information security, covering people, processes, and technology. For hospitals in both USA and India, ISO 27001 certification complements HIPAA (USA) and DPDPA (India) compliance by providing the management system structure that makes compliance sustainable.
ISO/IEC 42001:2023	Artificial Intelligence Management Systems, the world's first ISO standard specifically for AI management systems. Published in December 2023, this standard provides the framework for organizations to responsibly develop, deploy, and use AI systems, covering AI governance, risk management, performance evaluation, and continuous improvement. Hospital AI governance committees should be aware of ISO 42001 as the emerging global benchmark for AI management, and should consider alignment as AI programs mature.

13.4 HL7 FHIR: The Universal Language of Health Data

HL7 FHIR (Fast Healthcare Interoperability Resources) is the technical standard that is becoming the universal language for exchanging health information between systems, organizations, and countries. Understanding FHIR, at least at the conceptual level, is now essential for every healthcare leader, because it determines whether your systems can communicate with the rest of the healthcare ecosystem, and whether your AI tools can access the data they need.

What FHIR Is and Why It Matters

FHIR (pronounced 'fire') was developed by HL7 International to address a fundamental problem in healthcare: despite decades of effort, health information systems could not easily share data with each other. FHIR solves this by using modern web technology standards (REST APIs, JSON, XML) to define how health information should be represented and exchanged. Rather than proprietary data formats understood only by specific systems, FHIR defines standardized 'resources' such as Patient, Observation, Medication, Condition, and Diagnostic Report, that any FHIR-compliant system can read and write.

FHIR in Practice, What Healthcare Leaders Need to Know

- FHIR is mandated: the US 21st Century Cures Act requires EHR vendors to support FHIR R4 APIs, all major US EHR systems (Epic, Cerner, Meditech) now offer FHIR interfaces; India's ABDM has adopted FHIR as its national standard
- AI loves FHIR: FHIR APIs provide AI systems with structured, standardized access to patient data, eliminating custom integration work and enabling AI tools to work across multiple EHR platforms
- Patient data access: FHIR enables patients to access their own health records through mobile apps (Apple Health, Google Health) using standardized APIs, empowering patients and supporting health literacy
- Research and population health: FHIR enables de-identified patient data to be aggregated across institutions for research and population health analytics, the data foundation for AI training at scale
- Vendor evaluation: every EHR and AI vendor must support FHIR R4, verify this in contracts and conduct technical validation before procurement
- SMART on FHIR: the authorization framework that allows third-party apps (including AI tools) to securely access EHR data through FHIR APIs, enables the AI app ecosystem that is transforming healthcare

SNOMED CT, LOINC, and ICD-10: The Clinical Terminology Standards

FHIR provides the transport mechanism for health data. Clinical terminology standards ensure that the data being transported has a consistent, unambiguous meaning. Three terminology standards are essential to understand:

- SNOMED CT (Systematized Nomenclature of Medicine, Clinical Terms): the most comprehensive clinical terminology system in the world, covering diseases, findings, procedures, body structures, and more. Used in EHR systems to encode clinical concepts with precision. AI systems trained on SNOMED-coded data can generalize across institutions because the clinical concepts are consistently represented.
- LOINC (Logical Observation Identifiers Names and Codes): the standard for identifying laboratory tests, clinical observations, and vital signs. A LOINC code for 'serum potassium' means the same thing in a hospital in Mumbai and a hospital in Houston, enabling AI models trained on laboratory data from one site to work reliably at another.
- ICD-10 (International Classification of Diseases, 10th Revision): the global standard for classifying diagnoses and health problems. Used in clinical documentation, billing, quality measurement, and AI training data. Consistent ICD-10 coding is essential for AI diagnostic and outcome prediction models to perform reliably.

13.5 GDPR and European Healthcare Regulations: The Global Privacy Gold Standard

The General Data Protection Regulation (GDPR), enforced by the European Union since May 2018, is the most comprehensive personal data protection law in the world, and its influence extends far beyond Europe's borders. India's Digital Personal Data Protection Act (DPDPA) was modelled on GDPR principles. The US is actively debating federal privacy legislation that draws on GDPR frameworks. And any hospital in India or the United States that treats European patients, partners with European research institutions, or processes data of EU residents must understand and comply with GDPR.

For healthcare AI specifically, GDPR contains provisions that are more demanding than either HIPAA or the DPDPA, particularly around automated decision-making, the right to explanation, and the requirement for Data Protection Impact Assessments. Understanding GDPR is not merely a compliance exercise for international-facing institutions: it is a window into the direction that global AI regulation is moving, and a preview of what every country's health data regulations are likely to require within the next decade.

GDPR, Healthcare and AI Provisions at a Glance
Full Name: General Data Protection Regulation (EU) 2016/679, enforceable since May 25, 2018; applies to all processing of EU residents' personal data regardless of where the processor is located
Health Data Classification: Health data is classified as 'Special Category Data', the highest protection tier. Processing requires explicit consent OR another specific lawful basis (vital interests, public health, research)
Eight Patient Rights: Right to access; right to rectification; right to erasure ('right to be forgotten'); right to restriction; right to data portability; right to object; right not to be subject to automated decision-making; right to information
Right to Explanation (Article 22): Individuals have the right not to be subject to decisions based solely on automated processing, including AI, that significantly affects them. This directly governs clinical AI decision-making and requires explainable AI in clinical settings
Data Protection Impact Assessment (DPIA): Mandatory for any AI system processing health data at large scale or making automated decisions with significant effects, effectively requiring formal risk assessment before deploying clinical AI
Data Protection Officer (DPO): Hospitals and health systems processing health data at scale must appoint a qualified DPO, responsible for GDPR compliance including AI system oversight
Cross-Border Data Transfer: Transferring EU patient data outside the EU requires either adequacy decision, Standard Contractual Clauses, or Binding Corporate Rules, critical for Indian IT companies processing EU health data
Penalties: Up to 4% of global annual turnover or €20 million (whichever is higher) for serious violations, among the largest regulatory penalties in any sector globally

GDPR Article 22: The Right Not to Be Profiled by Algorithms Alone

Of all GDPR's provisions, Article 22 has the most direct and profound implications for healthcare AI governance. It establishes that individuals have the right not to be subject to decisions based solely on automated processing, including profiling, that produces legal or similarly significant effects concerning them.

In healthcare, a clinical decision about diagnosis, treatment, or a care plan clearly qualifies as a 'significantly significant effect.' This means that under GDPR, a hospital cannot allow an AI system to make or solely determine a clinical decision about an EU patient, there must always be meaningful human review and the ability for the patient to request human intervention. This requirement is not just ethically correct; it is legally mandatory for EU patients and represents the direction of global regulation.

This is why the principle established in Chapter 4, AI supports decisions, it never makes them, is not merely an ethical preference. It is, for European patients, a legal right. And it is the principle that every world-class hospital should apply to every patient, regardless of their nationality.

The EU AI Act 2024: The World's First Comprehensive AI Law

The European Union AI Act, passed in 2024, represents a historic milestone: the world's first comprehensive legal framework specifically governing artificial intelligence across all sectors, including healthcare. While it applies directly only within the EU, its global influence, like GDPR before it, is already shaping AI regulation in countries around the world, including discussions in India and the United States.

Risk Level	Definition	Healthcare AI Examples	Key Obligations
UNACCEPTABLE (Prohibited)	AI systems posing unacceptable risks to fundamental rights, banned outright	Biometric categorization by sensitive characteristics; social scoring systems applied to patients	BANNED, no deployment permitted under any circumstances
HIGH RISK (Strictly regulated)	AI used in critical infrastructure, education, employment, essential services, biometrics, including most clinical AI	AI diagnostic tools; AI surgical robots; AI clinical decision support; patient risk stratification systems; AI for medical device use	Conformity assessment before deployment; human oversight mandatory; transparency requirements; bias monitoring; registration in EU database; incident reporting
LIMITED RISK (Transparency required)	AI systems interacting with humans where transparency is needed	AI chatbots for patient communication; AI-generated patient education content; symptom checkers; AI-drafted discharge summaries	Must disclose that patient is interacting with AI; content generated by AI must be labeled as such
MINIMAL RISK (No specific obligations)	AI with minimal risk, most AI-enabled tools not making decisions about individuals	AI-powered spam filters; AI medical billing optimization; AI supply chain tools; AI for hospital energy management	No mandatory requirements, but voluntary codes of conduct encouraged

The EU AI Act's classification of most clinical AI as High Risk, with mandatory conformity assessment, human oversight, bias monitoring, and incident reporting, directly mirrors the governance framework recommended in this book. For healthcare leaders in India and the United States, the EU AI Act is not just a European compliance concern: it is a preview of the global regulatory direction and the strongest possible justification for building robust AI governance from the start.

CE Marking: European Medical Device Certification

For hospitals in India that treat European medical tourism patients, partner with European research institutions, or aspire to export AI-powered medical technologies, CE Marking, the European medical device certification, is an important credential to understand. The EU Medical Device Regulation (MDR 2017/745) governs CE Marking for medical devices, including AI-based SaMD (Software as a Medical Device).

CE Marking for AI medical devices requires: clinical evaluation demonstrating safety and performance; conformity assessment by a Notified Body (for class IIa and above); post-market surveillance; and, for AI/ML devices, specific attention to transparency, human oversight, and robustness requirements. The MDR also introduced the concept of 'legacy devices', AI systems already on the market that must be recertified under the new regulation.

GDPR and EU Regulations, What Indian and US Hospitals Must Do Today

- Identify EU patient population: understand how many EU residents you treat, whether online or in-person, if any, GDPR applies to their data
- Review vendor agreements: ensure any cloud provider, AI vendor, or IT partner processing EU patient data has signed Standard Contractual Clauses (SCCs), the EU-approved mechanism for international data transfer
- Assess AI systems against Article 22: for every AI system influencing clinical decisions about EU patients, confirm human oversight is real and documented, not just claimed

- Conduct Data Protection Impact Assessments (DPIAs): for any AI system processing EU health data at scale, DPIA is mandatory and must be documented
- Appoint or designate DPO responsibility: if processing EU health data at scale, a qualified Data Protection Officer must be designated and empowered
- Monitor EU AI Act implementation: high-risk healthcare AI compliance obligations begin in 2026, hospitals with EU-connected AI programs should begin gap assessment now
- Use GDPR as the quality benchmark: even for non-EU patients, GDPR's eight data rights and DPIA requirements represent best-practice data governance that any world-class institution should aspire to

13.6 Global Medical Education Accreditation: World-Class Standards for Training Doctors

Medical education accreditation defines the quality standards that medical colleges must meet to produce graduates who are competent, safe, and fit to practice. These standards, while administered nationally, are internationally benchmarked through the World Federation for Medical Education (WFME), whose recognition framework enables medical graduates to practice and pursue further training across international borders.

For Bhagyoday Hospital and Medical College, and for every institution aspiring to world-class medical education, understanding how Indian standards compare to global benchmarks is essential. It reveals both the minimum that must be met and the aspiration that separates good medical colleges from truly excellent ones.

Country	Body	Key Standards	AI/Digital Mandate
India NMC	Graduate Medical Education Regulations; CBME curriculum; NEXT exit exam; minimum infrastructure standards; faculty ratios	CBME includes health informatics; AI literacy not yet mandated but CBME framework accommodates it; digital skills increasingly expected	Primary compliance framework: CBME adoption with AI integration positions Bhagyoday ahead of peers
USA LCME	Liaison Committee on Medical Education, accredits all MD-granting programs; 12 standards covering mission, governance, faculty, students,	Medical Informatics in curriculum; evidence-based medicine; health systems science, AI literacy increasingly expected by residency programs	Benchmark for curriculum rigour and outcome measurement; LCME standards guide Bhagyoday's global-calibre curriculum design

	curriculum, facilities		
USA ACGME	Accreditation Council for Graduate Medical Education, accredits residency and fellowship programs; Milestones framework defines competency progression	Clinical Informatics as a formal ACGME sub-specialty; digital health tools in residency competency frameworks; AI decision support in training	Model for competency-based residency training; Bhagyoday postgraduate programs should align with the ACGME milestone framework
UK GMC	General Medical Council, Tomorrow's Doctors framework; Outcome for Graduates defines what all UK medical graduates must be able to do	Digital literacy and data skills now explicit in GMC Outcomes for Graduates (2018 onward); telehealth and AI clinical decision tools	GMC's explicit digital literacy outcomes serve as a global benchmark for what Bhagyoday graduates should achieve
Australia AMC	Australian Medical Council, Standards for Assessment and Accreditation of Primary Medical Programs; an international benchmark adopted by many Asian institutions	AMC standards include health informatics and evidence-based practice; digital health integration in the curriculum increasingly assessed	AMC standards valued by Indian institutions with international recognition ambitions; a useful benchmark for WFME alignment
Global WFME	World Federation for Medical Education, Basic Medical Education standards;	WFME standards increasingly reference digital health and health informatics as standard curriculum components	WFME recognition is the ultimate global credential, NMC alignment with WFME standards ensures Bhagyoday graduates are globally portable

	WFME recognition enables graduate cross-border portability and training rights		

The Dual Accreditation Model: Hospital + Medical College Together

Institutions like Bhagyoday, which are simultaneously hospitals and medical colleges, face a unique governance challenge and opportunity: they must satisfy two parallel accreditation frameworks, NABH for the hospital, NMC for the medical college, while building the integrated learning environment that makes them genuinely better than institutions operating either element separately.

The world's best academic medical centres, Mayo Clinic, Johns Hopkins, AIIMS Delhi, Christian Medical College Vellore, demonstrate that this integration, when done well, creates institutions where clinical excellence and educational excellence reinforce each other continuously. The hospital provides a clinical environment where students learn from real cases. The medical college creates a culture of inquiry, evidence-based practice, and continuous learning that elevates the clinical standards of the hospital. Each makes the other better.

For Bhagyoday, this integration is built into the institutional design: every clinical department is simultaneously a teaching department. Every improvement project is a learning opportunity for students. Every AI system is both a clinical tool and an educational one. This is not incidental; it is the deliberate design of an institution that takes both its clinical mission and its educational mission equally seriously.

Dual Accreditation Readiness, Hospital (NABH) and Medical College (NMC) Alignment Points

- Patient safety culture: both NABH and NMC CBME require demonstrated safety culture, safety teaching to students and safety management in the hospital reinforce each other
- Quality improvement: NABH CQI standards and NMC's research and quality expectations align, student improvement projects contribute to hospital quality outcomes
- Faculty development: NMC requires qualified, trained faculty; NABH requires trained clinical staff, joint faculty development programs satisfy both requirements efficiently
- Infection control and clinical environment: NMC requires adequate clinical training environment; NABH requires infection control standards, high NABH standards create better teaching environments
- Digital health infrastructure: NMC CBME health informatics requirements and NABH information management standards both require digital infrastructure, one investment serves both
- Ethics and patient rights: NMC AETCOM and NABH patient rights standards both require explicit ethics culture, ethics teaching and ethics governance reinforce each other
- Documentation and records: NMC requires clinical case documentation for student teaching; NABH requires complete clinical records for quality, the same records serve both purposes

13.7 Building Globally Informed, Locally Adapted Systems

The relationship between global standards and local practice is not one of simple compliance; it is one of informed adaptation. Global standards define the framework and the benchmarks. Local leaders adapt and apply them in ways that serve their specific patient population, cultural context, resource environment, and institutional maturity.

A hospital in rural Gujarat implementing NABH standards is doing something different from a hospital in Houston implementing Joint Commission standards, different patient population, different resources, different regulatory environment, different cultural context. But both are applying the same underlying quality principles: define what good care looks like, measure current performance, identify gaps, implement improvements, monitor results, and improve again. The global standards make this learning portable across contexts, so that a quality improvement approach proven in one country can be adapted and applied in another.

This is precisely the model of this book: drawing on the best quality management thinking from global industry and healthcare, the most rigorous regulatory frameworks from the United States and India, and the most powerful AI capabilities emerging globally, and synthesizing them into a practical framework for the world-class hospital, wherever in the world that hospital is being built.

★ KEY TAKEAWAYS

13. WHO's Global Patient Safety Action Plan and AI Ethics guidelines provide the global framework that every hospital AI governance program should align with.
14. ISO 9001 (quality management), ISO 13485 (medical devices), ISO 27001 (information security), and ISO 42001 (AI management) are the global standards that complement national accreditation requirements.
15. HL7 FHIR is the universal language of health data, every EHR and AI vendor must support it; it is the technical foundation for interoperability and AI data access.
16. GDPR is the world's gold standard for patient data privacy, its eight rights, Article 22 (right not to be profiled by AI alone), and DPIA requirements directly govern AI deployment for EU patients and set the global direction.
17. The EU AI Act 2024 classifies most clinical AI as high-risk, requiring conformity assessment, human oversight, bias monitoring, and incident reporting. This is the global regulatory future every hospital should prepare for now.
18. NMC's CBME framework is India's modern medical education standard, institutions integrating AI literacy within CBME are ahead of peers and aligned with global expectations.

19. Global medical education accreditation bodies, LCME, ACGME (USA), GMC (UK), AMC (Australia), WFME (Global), provide the international benchmarks that world-class Indian medical colleges should measure themselves against.
20. Dual accreditation institutions (hospital + medical college) create compounding excellence, clinical standards elevate teaching; teaching culture elevates clinical practice. One investment serves both missions.

▶ COMING NEXT

Chapter 14, the final and most important chapter of Part 4, addresses the most important and most complex dimension of AI in healthcare: ethics and governance. How do we ensure that AI serves all patients equally, that accountability is maintained, that bias is detected and corrected, and that the human values that define healthcare are preserved in an AI-integrated world?

Chapter 14

AI Ethics & Governance

Ethical Use, Bias and Fairness, Accountability, and the AI Ethics Committee Framework

> *"The measure of intelligence is the ability to change. The measure of wisdom is knowing which things must never change."*
>
> **Albert Einstein in healthcare AI, intelligence changes with every model update; wisdom protects the values that must remain constant.**

14.1 Introduction: Why Ethics Is the Most Important Chapter in This Book

Every chapter in this book describes how AI can make healthcare better, faster diagnoses, earlier detection of deterioration, more efficient operations, better quality measurement, and more equitable access to world-class care. The promise is real. The evidence is compelling. The opportunity is extraordinary.

And yet, AI can also make healthcare worse. Worse for patients who receive biased predictions because their demographic group was underrepresented in training data. Worse for clinicians who are deskilled by over-reliance on algorithmic recommendations. Worse for communities whose data is used without consent to train commercial AI systems. Worse for society if accountability becomes so diffused across humans and algorithms that no one can be held responsible when things go wrong.

The difference between AI that helps and AI that harms is not primarily a technical difference. It is an ethical and governance difference. It is determined by the decisions leaders make about how AI is designed, validated, deployed, monitored, and governed, and by whether those decisions are made with genuine commitment to the values that healthcare has always claimed as its own: beneficence, non-maleficence, justice, and respect for persons.

This chapter gives healthcare leaders the ethical framework, the governance structures, and the practical tools to ensure that AI in their institutions serves patients rather than harming them, and that the promise of AI is realized in ways that are worthy of the trust patients place in healthcare.

14.2 Foundational Ethics Principles: Applied to Healthcare AI

The four principles of biomedical ethics: developed by Beauchamp and Childress and known as 'principlism', have guided clinical ethics for decades. These same four principles, properly applied to AI, provide the ethical foundation for AI governance in healthcare.

1	**BENEFICENCE, AI must do good** **Definition:** The obligation to act in the best interest of patients, to actively promote their health and well-being. **In Healthcare AI:** Every AI system deployed in clinical settings must demonstrate that it improves patient outcomes, reduces harm, or enhances the quality of care. Deploying AI that has not been validated to benefit patients, even if it appears technically impressive, violates beneficence. **Leadership Action:** *Require clinical evidence of benefit before deployment. Every AI system must show measurable improvement in at least one patient outcome metric in a validated study population similar to yours.*
2	**NON-MALEFICENCE, AI must not harm** **Definition:** The obligation to avoid causing harm, 'first, do no harm' in the Hippocratic tradition. **In Healthcare AI:** AI systems can cause harm through inaccurate predictions, biased recommendations, alert fatigue that causes real alerts to be missed, deskilling of clinicians, and erosion of the patient-

provider relationship. Each of these harms must be actively monitored and mitigated.

Leadership Action: *Conduct pre-deployment harm assessment for every AI system. Define specific harm scenarios and monitoring metrics. Establish clear criteria for AI system suspension when harm thresholds are exceeded.*

3

JUSTICE, AI must be fair and equitable

Definition: The obligation to treat all patients fairly, distributing the benefits and burdens of AI equitably across all patient populations.

In Healthcare AI: AI systems trained on data that underrepresents certain populations, racial minorities, women, elderly patients, patients with disabilities, rural patients, will perform worse for those populations. This is not a technical glitch. It is an injustice that perpetuates and amplifies existing healthcare disparities.

Leadership Action: *Mandatory bias auditing for every AI system before deployment and quarterly thereafter. If an AI performs significantly worse for any demographic subgroup, it must not be deployed until the bias is corrected.*

4

AUTONOMY, AI must respect patient rights

Definition: The obligation to respect patients' right to make informed decisions about their own care, including their right to know how AI is used in their care.

In Healthcare AI: Patients have the right to know when AI is involved in decisions about their care, to understand how AI recommendations are generated, and to request human review of AI-supported decisions. Deploying AI without patient awareness violates the principle of informed consent.

Leadership Action: *Develop patient-facing AI disclosure language. Update informed consent processes to include AI use. Establish a patient's right to request AI-free care pathways where clinically feasible.*

14.3 Bias and Fairness in Healthcare AI: Understanding the Problem

Bias in AI is not hypothetical; it is documented, consequential, and widespread in healthcare AI systems. Understanding the sources of bias and the mechanisms for detecting and correcting them is one of the most important competencies a healthcare AI leader can develop.

Sources of Bias in Healthcare AI

- Historical data bias: AI models trained on historical patient data inherit the biases embedded in that data, including the documented disparities in how different patient populations have been diagnosed, treated, and monitored. A model trained on data from a healthcare system that historically undertreated pain in Black patients will learn to underpredict pain in Black patients.
- Sampling bias: models trained on data from academic medical centers, urban hospitals, or specific geographic regions may perform poorly when deployed in community hospitals, rural settings, or different demographic contexts. A model trained predominantly on male patients may miss disease presentations more common in women.
- Label bias: AI labels are created by human experts, and human expert judgment can carry bias. A diagnostic AI trained on radiologist annotations will inherit any systematic differences in how radiologists interpret images for different patient populations.
- Proxy variable bias: AI models sometimes use variables that appear neutral but serve as proxies for race or socioeconomic status, ZIP code as a proxy for race, insurance status as a proxy for income. Models using these variables can amplify structural inequities.
- Feedback loop bias: when AI recommendations influence clinical decisions, and those decisions generate the outcomes on which the AI is subsequently retrained, bias can be amplified over successive model generations.

The Bias Auditing Protocol, Minimum Requirements for Every Healthcare AI System

- Demographic subgroup analysis: measure AI performance (sensitivity, specificity, PPV, NPV) separately for every available demographic subgroup: age, gender, race/ethnicity, insurance status, language
- Disparity threshold: define an acceptable performance gap threshold (e.g., no more than 5% difference in sensitivity between demographic groups), any AI exceeding this threshold is not approved for deployment
- Intersectional analysis: examine performance at the intersection of demographic variables (e.g., elderly Black women, non-English-speaking patients), disparities often emerge most clearly at intersections
- Quarterly re-auditing: bias is not static, patient populations change, clinical practices evolve, and AI performance can drift. Re-audit every AI system quarterly and after any model update
- Corrective action protocol: when bias is detected, define and implement a corrective action plan, which may include model retraining, threshold adjustment, or system suspension pending correction
- Bias audit documentation: all bias audit results, including subgroup performance data and corrective actions, must be documented and available to the AI governance committee and, where appropriate, to the public

14.4 Accountability: Who Is Responsible When AI Is Involved?

The question of accountability in AI-assisted healthcare is one of the most difficult and most important questions in the field. When an AI system contributes to a patient harm event, a missed diagnosis, a delayed treatment, a biased recommendation, who is responsible?

The answer, in both US and Indian legal and ethical frameworks, is clear: the human clinician who made the final decision is responsible. AI is a tool. Like a stethoscope, a laboratory result, or a radiology read, AI provides information that a clinician uses to make decisions. The clinician who uses that information is accountable for the clinical decision, regardless of what the AI recommended.

This principle of human accountability is not merely a legal technicality. It is the ethical foundation for the appropriate use of AI in healthcare. It means that clinicians cannot delegate their judgment to algorithms, they must engage critically with AI outputs, maintain the clinical knowledge to evaluate AI recommendations, and accept responsibility for the decisions they make with AI assistance.

For healthcare institutions, accountability operates at a different level: the institution is responsible for selecting, validating, monitoring, and governing the AI systems it deploys. An institution that deploys an unvalidated AI system, fails to monitor it for performance drift, and does not train its staff to use it safely cannot defend itself behind 'the algorithm made the decision.'

AI Vendor Accountability	Hospital Institutional Accountability	Clinician Individual Accountability
• Transparent disclosure of training data, model architecture, and validation methodology • Accurate performance claims, including subgroup performance, not just overall metrics • Ongoing support and maintenance,	• Pre-deployment validation on the local patient population • AI governance committee oversight of all deployed systems • Staff training to the appropriate level for each AI system • Continuous monitoring of AI performance with defined	• Maintain clinical knowledge sufficient to evaluate AI recommendations • Engage critically with AI outputs, do not blindly follow algorithms • Document clinical reasoning when overriding AI recommendations • Report AI performance concerns through established channels

model updates, performance monitoring, regulatory changes • Adverse event reporting, notifying hospital customers when performance issues are identified • ISO 13485 certification and FDA clearance / CDSCO registration as applicable • Clear contractual liability framework including indemnification provisions	response protocols • Incident management for AI-related adverse events • Annual review and recertification of all AI systems • Board-level reporting on AI performance and safety	• Complete required AI literacy and system-specific training • Maintain human communication with patients about AI use in their care

14.5 The AI Ethics Committee: Structure and Function

Every healthcare institution deploying AI in clinical settings should establish a formal AI Ethics Committee, a cross-functional governance body responsible for ensuring that AI systems are evaluated, deployed, monitored, and governed according to the ethical principles and accountability frameworks described in this chapter.

The AI Ethics Committee is not the same as the IT steering committee, and it is not the same as the quality committee, though it works closely with both. It is a distinct governance body with a specific mandate: to ensure that AI serves patients and healthcare workers in ways that are ethical, equitable, accountable, and aligned with the institution's values.

AI Ethics Committee, Structure and Mandate
Composition: Chief Medical Officer (chair); Chief Information Officer; Chief Nursing Officer; Patient Safety Director; Clinical department representatives (rotating); Bioethicist or clinical ethics expert; Legal counsel; Patient/community representative; Data scientist / AI technical expert
Meeting Frequency: Monthly for ongoing governance; ad hoc for urgent AI-related safety or ethics concerns; annual comprehensive review of all AI systems
Pre-Deployment Review: Every new AI system must receive Committee approval before clinical deployment, clinical evidence review, bias audit results, governance plan, staff training plan, patient disclosure approach
Ongoing Monitoring: Monthly performance dashboard review; quarterly bias audit results; annual system recertification; review of all AI-related adverse events or near-misses
Policy Authority: The Committee has the authority to approve, modify, pause, or terminate any AI system deployment, decisions documented with rationale and communicated to affected clinical teams
Reporting: Reports to Board Quality Committee quarterly; provides annual AI governance report to hospital leadership; maintains AI system registry accessible to clinical staff
Documentation: AI system registry (all deployed systems, their validation status, performance data, governance plan); meeting minutes; decision records; incident reports; annual governance report

14.6 Transparency and Explainability: The Patient's Right to Understand

Transparency in AI means that patients, clinicians, and the public can understand how AI systems are being used in healthcare and what the basis for AI recommendations is. Explainability means that the specific output of an AI system, this alert, this prediction, this recommendation, can be explained in terms that a clinician can evaluate and a patient can understand.

Both are ethical requirements. A patient who learns that an AI system influenced a major clinical decision about their care has the right to ask: what did the AI consider? How confident was it? What would have happened if the AI had said something different? A clinician who receives an AI alert has the professional obligation to understand why it fired, not just what it recommends.

'Black box' AI, systems that generate outputs without any explainable basis, is ethically unacceptable in clinical settings where patients can be harmed by incorrect recommendations and clinicians are accountable for the decisions they make. This does not mean that every AI system must be a simple linear model, it means that every AI system deployed in clinical settings must have a mechanism for explaining its outputs at the level of clinical reasoning, even if the underlying model is complex.

AI Transparency Requirements, For Patients, Clinicians, and Leadership

- For patients: written disclosure that AI is used in their care, what types of decisions AI supports, their right to ask about AI recommendations, and their right to request human review, provided in accessible language in their preferred language
- For clinicians: clear documentation of what data inputs drove a specific AI alert or recommendation; confidence intervals or probability scores where available; known performance limitations for specific patient populations; how to document disagreement with AI recommendations
- For clinical leaders: monthly performance dashboard showing sensitivity, specificity, alert fatigue rates, override rates, and outcome data for every deployed AI system, with trend analysis and comparison to benchmark
- For governance: complete AI system registry with validation documentation, ongoing performance data, bias audit results, and incident reports, accessible to AI Ethics Committee and Board Quality Committee
- For the public: annual AI governance report describing what AI systems are used, how they are governed, and what the institution's AI ethics principles and commitments are, builds community trust in AI-integrated care

14.7 Real-World Reflection: Building the AI Ethics Framework at Bhagyoday

At Bhagyoday Hospital and Medical College, the AI Ethics Committee was established before the first AI system was deployed, not after a problem prompted its creation. This sequencing reflects a fundamental principle: ethics governance is a prerequisite for AI deployment, not an afterthought.

The Committee's first act was to develop the institution's AI Ethics Charter, a document that states, in plain language, the institution's commitments to patients, staff, and community regarding AI. The Charter is publicly available, reviewed annually, and used as the basis for evaluating every AI deployment decision. It has been translated into Gujarati and is available in the patient information provided at registration.

The Committee's bias auditing protocol is one of the most rigorous in any Indian healthcare institution: every AI system is audited quarterly against six demographic dimensions, with results reported to the Board and published in the annual AI governance report. When the institution's sepsis prediction AI was found in its first bias audit to show lower sensitivity for elderly female patients than for the general population, the Committee suspended the system, worked with the vendor on model recalibration, and did not redeploy until two consecutive audits showed equitable performance.

That decision, to suspend a system that was helping the majority of patients because it was not helping all patients equally, is the clearest expression of what AI ethics looks like in practice. Not in theory. In a real hospital, with real patients, making a real decision that was difficult and costly and absolutely right.

The medical students who train at Bhagyoday observe this governance in action. They attend AI Ethics Committee meetings as observers. They study the AI Ethics Charter as part of their professional formation. They graduate understanding not only how to use AI but how to govern it, and why that governance is as important as the technology itself.

★ KEY TAKEAWAYS

21. The four bioethics principles, Beneficence, Non-maleficence, Justice, Autonomy, provide the ethical framework for every AI deployment decision in healthcare.
22. Bias in healthcare AI is documented and consequential, sources include historical data bias, sampling bias, label bias, and proxy variable bias. Mandatory bias auditing is non-negotiable.
23. Human accountability is never displaced by AI, the clinician is responsible for decisions made with AI assistance; the institution is responsible for the AI systems it deploys.
24. The AI Ethics Committee is the governance mechanism that makes ethical AI real, with defined composition, authority, pre-deployment review, ongoing monitoring, and public reporting.
25. Transparency and explainability are ethical requirements, patients have the right to know when and how AI influences their care; clinicians have the right to understand why AI generated specific outputs.
26. WHO's six AI ethics principles: autonomy, well-being, transparency, accountability, inclusiveness, sustainability, are the global framework every AI Ethics Committee should align with.
27. Ethics governance is a prerequisite, not an afterthought, establish the AI Ethics Committee before the first AI system is deployed, not after the first problem occurs.

▶ COMING NEXT

Part 5 of this book turns to the transformation of medical education, how AI is changing how we teach and learn medicine, how to build world-class medical education systems for the 21st century, and how to develop the future doctors and faculty who will lead the AI-integrated healthcare systems we are building today.

PART FIVE

World-Class Medical Education

Rethinking how we teach, learn, and develop the doctors and faculty who will lead healthcare's AI-integrated future

Chapter 15

Rethinking Medical Education

The Gaps in Today's System, the Demands of Tomorrow, and the Vision of World-Class Medical Training

> *"The function of education is to teach one to think intensively and to think critically. Intelligence plus character; that is the goal of true education."*
>
> **Martin Luther King Jr., a standard that every medical college must aspire to, and very few currently achieve.**

15.1 Introduction: Why Medical Education Must Be Rethought Now

Medical education is in crisis. It is a quiet crisis that rarely makes headlines but is felt every day by patients, physicians, and the communities healthcare systems serve. The crisis has multiple dimensions: a curriculum designed for a world of certainty being delivered to students entering a world of rapid change; a teaching approach that rewards memorization over reasoning; a system that produces technically trained doctors who are sometimes poorly prepared for the human complexity of clinical practice; and a near-total absence of preparation for the AI-integrated healthcare environment these students will spend their entire careers working in.

This is not a criticism of individual educators or institutions. It is a structural observation about a system that has changed less in the past 50 years than almost any other professional education in the world. The fundamental structure of medical education, two years of pre-clinical science followed by two years of clinical clerkships, assessed by written examinations, supervised by senior physicians who themselves trained under the same system, was established in the early 20th century and has remained largely intact.

Meanwhile, the world has transformed. The medical knowledge base has expanded beyond any individual's capacity to retain fully. Artificial intelligence is performing diagnostic tasks with accuracy that equals or exceeds trained specialists. Genomic medicine is personalizing treatment at the molecular level. Global pandemics are reshaping public health. And the patients whom doctors serve are more informed, more demanding, and more diverse than ever before.

Evidence from leading institutions suggests that effective solutions are achievable. World-class medical education systems, in Singapore, in the Netherlands, in Canada, in select institutions across India and the United States, have demonstrated that transformation is possible. The principles are clear and the evidence is robust, and the technology to support transformation is available. What remains is the leadership will to implement it.

This chapter examines the gaps in current medical education, the demands of the 21st-century healthcare environment, and the vision of world-class medical training that every institution, including Bhagyoday, must work toward.

15.2 Current Gaps in Medical Education: An Honest Diagnosis

Effective improvement begins with an honest diagnosis. Before we can build the medical education system the future requires, we must name clearly what the current system is failing to provide.

Curriculum Gaps	Pedagogy Gaps	Values & Culture Gaps
• Overemphasis on memorization of facts that AI can retrieve in seconds	• Lecture-dominant teaching, passive learning, poor retention	• Communication skills and empathy taught by lecture, not practice • Patient-centered care as

• Insufficient training in clinical reasoning under uncertainty • Little to no AI literacy, digital health, or health informatics • Quality improvement and patient safety not adequately taught • Research methodology taught theoretically, not practically • Health economics, healthcare systems, and leadership largely absent • Interprofessional education minimal, doctors train in silos • Community medicine disconnected from clinical training	• Insufficient simulation and skills lab training before patient contact • Competency-based progression not consistently implemented • Formative feedback rare, students learn at summative exams • Problem-based and case-based learning underutilized • Technology-enhanced learning largely absent or ad hoc • Student wellbeing is poorly supported, burnout rates alarming • Little structured mentorship beyond informal relationships	philosophy, not embedded in daily teaching • Ethics education sporadic rather than integrated throughout • Hierarchy culture suppresses questions and mistakes learning • No formal preparation for leadership or system change • Cultural competency for diverse patient populations inadequate • Professionalism is modeled inconsistently by faculty • AI ethics and digital professionalism not addressed

The India-Specific Context

In India, medical education faces additional structural challenges that are specific to its scale and developmental context. With over 700 medical colleges producing approximately 90,000 MBBS graduates annually, quality is highly variable. The top 50 institutions, the IIMSes, AIIMS, CMC Vellore, and leading private medical colleges, produce graduates of genuinely world-class quality. The bottom quartile of institutions, however, produces graduates with serious gaps in clinical competency that have direct patient safety implications.

The root causes in India include: infrastructure inadequacy in many colleges (insufficient clinical exposure due to inadequate patient volumes or bed strength), faculty shortages, particularly in specialist disciplines, examination systems that reward rote learning over clinical reasoning, and limited exposure to quality management, research methodology, and digital health. NMC's CBME reforms are addressing many of these gaps systematically, but implementation quality varies dramatically across institutions.

The USA-Specific Context

In the United States, medical education operates through an extremely well-regulated system with high average quality, but faces its own distinct challenges. The cost of medical education has become a crisis: the average US medical student graduates with over $200,000 in debt, which distorts career choices toward high-income specialties and away from primary care, rural medicine, and underserved communities. This financial distortion has profound implications for health equity.

US medical education is also grappling seriously with the integration of AI and digital health. The AAMC (Association of American Medical Colleges) has published AI competencies for medical students and physicians. Major medical schools, including Stanford, UCSF, and Harvard, are developing AI medicine curricula. ACGME residency programs are beginning to define AI-related competencies. The direction is clear; but implementation is uneven, and the pace needs to accelerate.

15.3 What 21st-Century Medical Education Must Develop

If the current system has gaps, what must the transformed system provide? The answer is not a longer list of topics to memorize; it is a fundamentally different model of what a medical graduate is equipped to do.

The 21st-century physician must be simultaneously: a skilled clinical diagnostician and decision-maker; a compassionate communicator who can navigate the most difficult human conversations with grace; a critical consumer of evidence, including AI-generated evidence; a quality improvement practitioner who can identify system failures and fix them; a digital health professional who can use, evaluate, and govern AI tools; a lifelong learner who continuously updates knowledge in an era of exponential medical advance; and a leader who can contribute to institutional and system transformation.

This is a more ambitious vision than any single curriculum currently fulfills. But it is the vision that every genuinely world-class medical education program is working toward.

The Seven Competencies of the World-Class 21st-Century Physician

- Clinical Excellence: deep, current, evidence-based clinical knowledge, applied with sound reasoning under uncertainty, not retrieved from memory alone
- Compassionate Communication: mastery of the art of patient communication, breaking bad news, shared decision-making, cultural sensitivity, digital communication, and family engagement
- Critical AI Literacy: ability to use, evaluate, interrogate, and govern AI clinical decision support, neither blindly trusting nor reflexively rejecting algorithmic recommendations
- Quality and Safety Leadership: understanding of quality improvement methodology, able to identify system failures, lead improvement projects, and contribute to safety culture
- Research and Evidence Mastery: ability to critically appraise clinical research, including AI-generated evidence, and to conduct and publish meaningful research

- Systems Thinking: understanding of healthcare systems, economics, policy, and leadership, able to function effectively as a change agent within complex institutions
- Lifelong Learning Discipline: a personal learning system that ensures knowledge remains current throughout a 30-40 year career, including regular AI and digital health upskilling

★ KEY TAKEAWAYS

1. Medical education is in quiet crisis, curriculum gaps, pedagogical failures, and values deficits are producing physicians inadequately prepared for the AI-integrated 21st century.
2. India's gaps include variable quality, examination systems rewarding memorization, and limited AI/digital health exposure, NMC's CBME is the reform framework, implementation quality is the variable.
3. USA's gaps include cost-driven specialty distortion and uneven AI curriculum integration, the AAMC AI competency framework is the emerging standard.
4. The 21st-century physician must master seven competencies: Clinical Excellence, Compassionate Communication, Critical AI Literacy, Quality Leadership, Research Mastery, Systems Thinking, and Lifelong Learning.

▶ COMING NEXT

Chapter 16 examines how AI is specifically transforming medical education, as a teaching tool, a simulation platform, a personalised learning engine, and a clinical training partner. The technology is available now. The question is how to deploy it to maximum educational effect.

Chapter 16

AI in Medical Education

How Artificial Intelligence Is Transforming How We Teach, Learn, Simulate, and Personalise the Journey to Becoming a Doctor

> *"Tell me, and I forget. Teach me, and I remember. Involve me, and I learn."*
>
> **Benjamin Franklin, whose 18th-century wisdom perfectly describes why AI-enabled active learning works so much better than passive lectures.**

16.1 Introduction: AI as the Most Powerful Educational Tool Ever Available

Medical education has always been limited by two constraints: the availability of expert teachers and the availability of learning opportunities. Great teachers are scarce; there are never enough of them to give every student the individual attention and feedback that optimal learning requires. And clinical learning opportunities are unpredictable, the right patient, with the right presentation, at the right stage of a student's training, does not always appear on schedule.

Artificial intelligence significantly reduces both constraints. An AI tutor is available 24 hours a day, consistently available and highly responsive, able to adapt its explanations to the exact level of understanding the student has demonstrated, and capable of providing immediate, specific, actionable feedback on every practice question, every simulated clinical encounter, and every submitted case analysis. An AI simulation platform can generate any clinical scenario, any physical examination finding, any laboratory result pattern, any imaging study, on demand, at any level of complexity, as many times as the student needs to achieve competency.

This is not merely a future possibility. These tools exist today and are being used in medical education programs around the world. This chapter examines the major categories of AI application in medical education, describes specific tools and platforms, and provides guidance for medical educators and institutional leaders on how to integrate AI into education programs effectively, ethically, and in alignment with CBME and global curriculum standards.

16.2 AI Tutoring and Adaptive Learning Systems

The most fundamental application of AI in medical education is personalized, adaptive tutoring, the ability to deliver learning content and assessment that automatically adjusts to each student's current level of knowledge, learning pace, and specific gaps.

Traditional medical education is largely undifferentiated: all students in a cohort receive the same lectures, the same reading assignments, and the same examinations. A student who has already mastered cardiovascular pharmacology sits through the same lecture as a student who is encountering the topic for the first time. A student who struggles with renal physiology receives no additional support between scheduled tutorials. This one-size-fits-all approach produces predictably uneven outcomes.

Adaptive AI learning systems change this fundamentally. They assess each student's current knowledge state, through formative questions, concept maps, and performance data, and then curate a personalized learning pathway that focuses time and attention on the specific gaps each student has, at the appropriate level and in the learning format best suited to them.

AI Tool / Platform	What It Does	Educational Application	Implementation Consideration
Amboss	Medical knowledge platform with AI-powered question bank and learning analytics, 60,000+ questions with spaced	USMLE and NMC NEXT preparation; clinical reasoning development; self-directed learning	Subscription cost; requires internet connectivity; content primarily US-oriented, supplementation with

	repetition and performance analytics	between teaching sessions	the Indian clinical context needed
Osmosis / Elsevier	AI-curated medical education content with video, visual mnemonics, and adaptive question banks, integrates with EHR systems for clinical learning	Pre-clinical science reinforcement; clinical clerkship preparation; spaced repetition for long-term retention	Strong visual learning support; EHR integration enables contextual learning at the point of care during clinical rotations
Aquifer	Virtual patient cases with branching clinical decision scenarios, evidence-based cases developed by US medical schools	Clinical reasoning development; diagnosis and management decision-making; CBME competency assessment	Excellent for clinical reasoning training; case library growing; faculty development needed for effective integration into the curriculum
Google MedPaLM / Claude	Large language model AI systems capable of answering clinical questions, explaining concepts, generating practice cases, and providing feedback on written work	On-demand concept explanation; practice case generation; essay and case report feedback; Socratic questioning for deeper learning	Requires critical evaluation skills. AI systems can generate plausible but incorrect outputs; must be taught as a decision-support tool, not an answer source; institutional AI literacy prerequisite
Anki with AI Integration	Spaced repetition flashcard system enhanced with AI content generation and performance-adaptive scheduling	Long-term retention of high-yield clinical facts; pharmacology, anatomy, and clinical signs; NEXT and USMLE preparation	Free platform; AI integration through third-party tools; requires faculty curation of card decks for India-specific content
Lecturio / Marrow	Comprehensive AI-powered question banks and video lecture platforms, Marrow, specifically	CBME-aligned content delivery; NEXT preparation; clinical case studies;	Marrow specifically calibrated to Indian NMC requirements; analytics allow faculty to identify cohort-level

	designed for NMC NEXT	performance analytics for faculty oversight	learning gaps proactively

16.3 Simulation and Virtual Training: Learning Without Risk to Patients

The fundamental ethical challenge in clinical medical education is that students must practice on patients, but patients have the right not to be the subjects of incompetent practice. This tension has always existed, and has always been managed through supervision: students practice under the watchful eye of experienced clinicians who can intervene before harm occurs. But supervision has limits; it is resource-intensive, inconsistently available, and cannot fully protect patients from the inherent risk of trainee practice.

AI-powered simulation changes this equation profoundly. Students can practice clinical procedures, diagnostic reasoning, emergency responses, and communication skills in simulated environments that provide realistic fidelity, immediate feedback, and zero risk to real patients. They arrive in clinical settings having already practiced the skill dozens or hundreds of times, with their errors occurring in simulation rather than on patients.

High-Fidelity Clinical Simulation

Modern clinical simulation centres deploy AI-enhanced mannequins that can simulate virtually any physiological state: cardiac arrest, respiratory failure, anaphylaxis, septic shock, obstetric emergencies, and pediatric critical illness. These mannequins respond to interventions, medications, airway management, chest compressions, with physiologically accurate responses generated by AI algorithms. A student performing a simulated rapid sequence intubation experiences the full procedural and decision-making complexity of the real procedure, without any risk to a real patient.

In India, NMC's CBME regulations now require simulation centre infrastructure as a component of medical college accreditation. This is the correct requirement, but compliance varies enormously between institutions. Bhagyoday's simulation centre is designed from inception as a core teaching facility, not a compliance checkbox, with a curriculum-integrated simulation program that mirrors the clinical training students receive in the wards.

Virtual Reality and AI-Powered Clinical Scenarios

Beyond physical mannequins, virtual reality (VR) and AI-generated clinical scenario platforms are creating entirely new categories of educational experience. VR anatomy platforms allow students to explore three-dimensional human anatomy at the resolution of individual structures, transforming a subject that has historically required cadaver dissection into an interactive, repeatable, visually rich learning experience. AI clinical scenario generators can create thousands of unique patient cases, varying presentation, demographics, comorbidities, and diagnostic complexity, giving students an essentially infinite library of practice cases.

Platforms like Touch Surgery (procedural skills), 3D4Medical (anatomy), and Anatomage (virtual dissection) are already in use in medical schools across the USA and, increasingly, in leading Indian institutions. The investment required is significant but increasingly competitive with the cost of traditional cadaver programs, and the educational return, in terms of engagement, retention, and transferable skill, is demonstrably superior for many learning objectives.

OSCE Preparation with AI: Objective Structured Clinical Examinations

The Objective Structured Clinical Examination (OSCE) is the gold standard for assessing clinical skills competency, and one of the most anxiety-inducing assessments in medical education. AI is transforming OSCE preparation in two important ways: AI-powered standardised patient simulators allow students to practice clinical encounters with AI-driven virtual patients that respond realistically to student communication, examination findings, and management decisions; and AI assessment tools can evaluate video recordings of student OSCE performance, providing structured feedback on communication, clinical reasoning, and procedural technique that previously required human expert review.

NMC's NEXT examination includes an OSCE component, making high-quality OSCE preparation an institutional imperative for every Indian medical college. AI-powered OSCE preparation platforms extend access to structured clinical skills practice to every student, regardless of the scheduling constraints of physical simulation facilities.

6.4 Personalised Learning: AI Meeting Every Student Where They Are

Perhaps the most transformative potential of AI in medical education is its ability to make genuinely personalised learning achievable at scale. Every student in a medical cohort is different: different prior knowledge, different learning style, different strengths and weaknesses, different pace of progress, different aspirations. Traditional medical education ignores most of this variation, every student gets the same curriculum, at the same pace, assessed by the same examination.

AI changes this by making it computationally feasible to track each student's learning trajectory with granular detail, identify specific knowledge gaps and skill deficits, recommend targeted learning activities to address those specific gaps, and adjust the pace and depth of curriculum delivery to match demonstrated readiness. This is not a luxury; it is the condition for genuinely competency-based education, in which students progress upon demonstrated mastery rather than upon time elapsed.

The Personalised Learning System, How AI Enables True Competency-Based Education

- Continuous formative assessment: AI-powered question banks and case platforms continuously assess student knowledge state, not just at scheduled examinations, but throughout every learning interaction

- Learning gap mapping: AI identifies each student's specific knowledge and skill gaps, not 'the student is weak in medicine' but 'this student has not demonstrated competency in heart failure management, diabetic emergencies, and acute kidney injury'
- Personalised learning recommendations: AI curates a specific learning pathway for each identified gap, the right content, at the right level, in the right format (video, reading, practice questions, simulation), in the right sequence
- Pace adaptation: AI tracks whether students are progressing at expected rates and flags those who are falling behind for faculty early intervention, enabling proactive support rather than reactive response to examination failure
- Strength amplification: AI identifies student strengths and interests and helps channel them, supporting the development of the unique professional identity that produces distinctive, excellent physicians rather than standardised graduates
- Faculty analytics: aggregate learning data across the cohort reveals curriculum-level gaps, if 40% of students are consistently failing questions on a specific topic, the curriculum, not the students, needs revision

16.5 AI for Teaching and Faculty Support

AI benefits not only students but also faculty, the teachers who are the heart of every great medical education program. Faculty members in medical colleges carry extraordinary burdens: clinical service, teaching, research, administration, and the continuing development of their own clinical and educational expertise. AI tools that reduce the administrative burden of teaching, without reducing the quality of the educational experience, free faculty to do what they do best: mentor, inspire, challenge, and model the values and practices of excellent medicine.

AI for Teaching Preparation	AI for Student Assessment	AI for Faculty Development
• Case generation: AI generates diverse patient case scenarios for PBL and TBL sessions, reducing faculty preparation time by 50-70% • Question bank development: AI generates and validates formative assessment questions aligned to learning objectives • Lecture enhancement: AI tools assist in designing active learning components, creating visual aids, and identifying up-to-date evidence • Feedback generation: AI provides structured written feedback on student submissions: faculty review and personalise before delivery	• Automated marking of objective questions with detailed performance analytics at individual and cohort level • AI-assisted evaluation of written case analyses: scoring for structure, clinical reasoning quality, and evidence use • OSCE performance analysis from video recordings, structured feedback on communication and procedural skills • Portfolio review support, AI flags patterns of strength and concern across longitudinal student portfolios	• Evidence-based teaching practice recommendations tailored to faculty's specific teaching assignments and student cohort • AI-powered peer observation tools, structured frameworks for observing and giving feedback on colleagues' teaching • Personal CPD tracking, AI monitors faculty continuing professional development against NMC/ACGME requirements • Research support, AI literature review, methodology advice, and manuscript preparation assistance • AI in my specialty: curated AI tool recommendations specific to each faculty member's

• Literature monitoring: AI tools track new evidence in faculty's specialty areas and flag relevant updates for curriculum inclusion	• Plagiarism and academic integrity detection, essential as AI content generation becomes widespread among students	clinical and teaching specialty

16.6 Critical AI Literacy: Teaching Students How to Use AI Responsibly

Perhaps the most important AI-related educational task is teaching medical students not just how to use AI tools, but how to use them critically, responsibly, and with appropriate skepticism. A physician who receives an AI diagnostic recommendation and accepts it without interrogation is not safer than the physician who has no AI; they are more dangerous, because they have the false confidence of algorithmic authority without the critical evaluation that clinical responsibility requires.

AI literacy education in medical school must cover: how AI systems work at a conceptual level, what training data means, what a false positive rate means, what model drift means; how to interrogate AI recommendations, what data drove this output, what is the confidence level, what demographic was this validated on; how to document AI involvement in clinical reasoning, the professional obligation to maintain transparent records of how decisions were made; how to report AI performance concerns, the institutional mechanisms for raising concerns about underperforming AI systems; and the ethical obligations of AI-era physicians, toward patients whose care is influenced by AI, toward the integrity of clinical data, and toward the fair and equitable use of AI across all patient populations.

This education cannot be delivered as a single module in the first year and can never be revisited. It must be woven throughout the curriculum, revisited at increasing levels of sophistication as students progress through clinical training, and modelled by faculty who themselves demonstrate critical AI use in their own clinical practice

★ KEY TAKEAWAYS

5. AI has the potential to become one of the most powerful educational tools available for medical education, providing infinite patient cases, adaptive personalization, immediate feedback, and 24/7 availability.
6. Adaptive AI learning platforms (Amboss, Osmosis, Aquifer, Marrow) personalize the learning pathway to each student's specific gaps, enabling genuine competency-based progression.
7. AI simulation, high-fidelity mannequins, VR anatomy, AI-generated clinical scenarios, AI OSCE preparation, allows students to achieve competency before practicing on real patients.
8. Personalized learning at scale is AI's most transformative educational capability, tracking every student's learning trajectory and curating targeted pathways to address specific gaps.
9. AI supports faculty too, in case preparation, formative assessment, cohort analytics, and personal development, freeing them to focus on mentorship and values formation.
10. Critical AI literacy is the most important AI-related educational task, students must learn to interrogate, not just use, AI recommendations in clinical settings.
11. The Bhagyoday model demonstrates AI integration done right: AI as a learning partner throughout the curriculum, with faculty oversight, critical evaluation, and always student reasoning as the final authority.

▶ COMING NEXT

Chapter 17 focuses on the students themselves, the future doctors being built by these educational systems. What specific qualities, competencies, and habits of mind must world-class medical education develop? How do we produce physicians who are technically excellent, deeply human, lifelong learners, and effective leaders?

Chapter 17

Building Future Doctors

Knowledge, Skills, Humanity, Decision-Making, Communication, and the Habit of Lifelong Learning

> *"The best doctor is the one who, when there is nothing to be done, does nothing, and when there is everything to be done, knows exactly what to do and how to do it with compassion."*
>
> **Adapted from Sir William Osler, the father of modern medicine, whose wisdom remains the most precise definition of the excellent physician.**

17.1 Introduction: What We Are Really Building

A medical college does not produce doctors. It creates the conditions in which young people with intelligence, commitment, and potential become doctors, through years of study, practice, mentorship, failure, growth, and ultimately, through thousands of encounters with human beings in their most vulnerable moments.

This distinction matters. It means that the responsibility of a medical educator is not to deliver a curriculum. It is to shape a person. A person who will, over a 30- to 40-year career, make decisions that affect millions of human lives. Who will sit with patients in moments of fear and uncertainty and need to be fully present, both technically competent and deeply human. Who will work in increasingly complex systems with AI tools, interprofessional teams, and quality governance frameworks, and need to navigate all of this without losing sight of the patient at the cen ter.

This chapter examines what world-class medical education must build in each student, the knowledge architecture that endures, the clinical skills that save lives, the communication abilities that build trust, the decision-making capacity that serves patients under uncertainty, and the learning habits that sustain excellence across an entire career.

17.2 Knowledge: Building the Right Foundation

The knowledge challenge in 21st-century medical education is not a shortage of content; it is a surplus. Some estimates suggest that the medical knowledge base doubles approximately every 73 days. No human being can hold all of it in memory. No curriculum can teach all of it. The question is not 'what do students need to know' but 'how should knowledge be structured so that it enables excellent clinical reasoning', and 'what do students need to know how to find, rather than simply know?'

World-class medical education builds knowledge in three layers: foundational science (the mechanisms that underlie disease and treatment, understanding, not memorization); core clinical knowledge (the essential facts, frameworks, and patterns that every physician needs immediately accessible for every clinical encounter; this is the high-yield core that must be genuinely learned); and navigational knowledge (knowing where to find the rest, how to search the literature, how to interpret systematic reviews, how to use clinical decision support tools including AI, how to consult specialists effectively).

The shift from a memorization-dominant to a reasoning-dominant knowledge model is not a lowering of standards; it is a raising of them. A physician who understands why metformin works in type 2 diabetes is far more capable of individualizing treatment than one who can recite its mechanism from memory without understanding its implications. Understanding enables adaptation. Memorization enables only reproduction.

17.3 The Year-by-Year Competency Journey: MBBS to Independent Practice

Building a physician takes time, and the progression from novice to competent clinician follows a predictable developmental trajectory that world-class education programs design their curriculum around. The following framework maps the competency milestones across the MBBS program and early postgraduate training:

Year	Focus	Knowledge	Skills	Attitude	AI Integration
Year 1	Foundations	Anatomy, physiology, biochemistry, mechanisms, not memorisation. Disease concepts introduced through clinical correlation	Clinical communication basics; history-taking introduction; simulation lab fundamentals; basic life support certified	Professional identity formation; patient-centered values introduction; AETCOM ethics foundation; healthcare system orientation	AI literacy introduction: what AI is, how it works in healthcare, how to use AI learning tools critically and responsibly
Year 2	Pathology & Pharmacology	Pathology, microbiology, pharmacology, linking mechanism to disease and treatment. Evidence-based medicine introduced	Clinical examination skills in simulation; structured history-taking on real patients with supervision; procedural skills lab	Informed consent practice; patient communication under supervision; team-based care introduction; error reporting culture	AI diagnostic tool awareness: how AI reads ECGs, X-rays, lab patterns; practice with AI case platforms; critical appraisal of AI outputs
Year 3	Clinical Entry	Medicine, surgery, pediatrics, OB/GYN, clinical presentation patterns, diagnostic frameworks, management principles	Clinical clerkships begin; supervised patient management; OSCE milestone assessment; procedural	Patient advocacy; difficult communication supervised; interprofessional team participation; quality improvement	AI in clinical clerkships: AI clinical decision support tools in supervised use; EHR AI alerts; structured reflection on AI

			competency in core skills	project begins	recommendations
Year 4	Clinical Consolidation	Specialty rotations; complex case management; research methodology; healthcare systems and leadership	Independent clinical reasoning with supervision; emergency simulations; research project design; leadership project	Independent professional identity; teaching junior students; quality improvement project completion; professional portfolio	AI governance participation: AI ethics committee observation; AI performance monitoring in clinical departments; AI literacy teaching to junior students
Internship	Supervised Independence	Applied clinical knowledge across all disciplines; continuing education habit established; NEXT preparation	First-call independent management; procedural independence in core skills; team leadership; handoff communication	Full professional responsibility; patient safety culture contribution; community medicine service; professional reflection	Full AI integration: independent use of validated AI tools with critical evaluation; AI incident reporting; mentoring medical students on AI use

17.4 Clinical Skills: The Art and Science of the Examination

Clinical skills, the ability to elicit a history, perform a physical examination, interpret investigations, and synthesise a clinical assessment, are the core technical competency of the physician. They are also the domain most threatened by two complementary risks: the risk of under-training (insufficient practice before patient contact) and the risk of technological substitution (using technology to bypass the clinical examination rather than enhance it).

World-class clinical skills education addresses both risks: through simulation training before patient contact, ensuring students arrive in clinical environments with practiced skills rather than learning on vulnerable patients; and through deliberate practice frameworks that maintain the clinical examination as a core skill even as AI diagnostic tools proliferate.

An ECG read by an AI algorithm is more accurate than most generalist physicians, but the physician who cannot read the ECG independently cannot evaluate whether the algorithm has made an error, cannot practice in settings where the AI is unavailable, and cannot teach the next generation. Clinical examination skills must be taught, practiced, assessed, and maintained, with AI as an enhancement, not a replacement.

Core Clinical Skills: Minimum Competency Standards for Every MBBS Graduate

- History-taking: structured, patient-centered, culturally sensitive history from patients across age groups and presentations, including digital/telemedicine history-taking
- Physical examination: complete systematic examination across all systems; targeted examination for focused clinical questions; examination adapted for pediatric, obstetric, and elderly patients
- Clinical reasoning: systematic differential diagnosis generation; evidence-based investigation ordering; risk stratification; treatment planning aligned to patient values and evidence
- Procedural skills: IV access, venepuncture, urinary catheterisation, nasogastric tube insertion, basic wound care, basic airway management, basic resuscitation, each certified in simulation before first patient use
- Investigations interpretation: ECG, chest X-ray, basic laboratory results (CBC, metabolic panel, urinalysis, arterial blood gas), independent interpretation with AI as secondary verification
- Emergency management: ABCDE approach, basic life support, ALS fundamentals, obstetric emergencies, pediatric emergencies, simulation-certified at each stage

- Clinical documentation: accurate, complete, legible clinical records, whether handwritten or electronic, with appropriate AI-assisted documentation tools used with clinical oversight
- Handover communication: structured SBAR handover; telephone consultations; referral letter writing; discharge summary preparation

17.5 Communication Skills: The Most Underestimated Clinical Competency

If a physician has the diagnostic acumen of Sherlock Holmes but cannot communicate a diagnosis, a treatment plan, or difficult news in a way that a patient can understand and act upon, their clinical excellence is substantially wasted. Communication is not a soft skill peripheral to medicine. It is the primary interface between clinical knowledge and patient benefit.

The evidence strongly supports this conclusion. Physicians with strong communication skills have patients who adhere better to treatment plans, who report higher satisfaction, who experience fewer adverse events from miscommunication, who are less likely to complain or litigate, and who have demonstrably better health outcomes on measured indicators. Communication training is, quite literally, patient safety training.

And yet, in most medical schools worldwide, communication skills receive a fraction of the curriculum time given to pharmacology or pathology. Students are exposed to communication theory in lectures and perhaps a handful of role-play exercises, without the deliberate practice and feedback that produce genuine competency.

World-class communication education uses a different model: repeated, structured practice with standardised patients (real or AI-simulated); video review with individualised feedback; progressive complexity across training years; and faculty who model exceptional communication in their own clinical practice and reflect on it explicitly with students.

Breaking Difficult News	Shared Decision-Making	Digital & Telemedicine Communication
• SPIKES protocol (Setting, Perception, Invitation, Knowledge, Empathy, Strategy), practiced in simulation with feedback • Delivering cancer diagnosis, terminal prognosis, unexpected fetal anomaly, sudden death notification • Cultural variation in communication preferences, when family is the primary interlocutor • When to pause, when to continue, how to manage silences • AI role: AI standardised patient for practice; AI sentiment analysis of communication recordings for feedback	• Eliciting patient values and preferences, not just informing, but genuinely engaging • Presenting risk and benefit information in formats patients can understand • Decision aids: paper, digital, and AI-generated personalised formats • When the patient's choice conflicts with clinical recommendation • AI role: AI generates personalised decision aids; AI risk communication tools calibrated to patient health literacy	• Video consultation etiquette, establishing rapport, managing examination limitations, maintaining privacy • Written communication: clear, jargon-free patient messages; EHR patient portal communication • AI-assisted communication, informing patients about AI use in their care; transparent AI disclosure • Cross-cultural and language-barrier communication, when to use AI translation tools • AI role: AI quality assessment of written patient communications; telemedicine simulation platforms

17.6 Decision-Making Under Uncertainty: The Essential Clinical Skill

Medicine is fundamentally a discipline of uncertainty. The textbook patient, whose symptoms fit neatly into a classic presentation, whose tests confirm the suspected diagnosis, and whose treatment follows the evidence-based protocol exactly, exists more often in examinations than in real clinical practice. Real patients are complex, atypical, contradictory, and frequently uncertain about their own symptoms. Real clinical decisions must often be made with incomplete information, time pressure, and significant consequences for error.

Teaching students to reason well under uncertainty, rather than to wait for certainty that never arrives, is one of the most important and most neglected tasks of medical education. It requires explicit teaching of cognitive frameworks for decision-making, deliberate exposure to ambiguous clinical scenarios in simulation and supervised practice, and reflection on the reasoning processes behind clinical decisions.

AI adds a new dimension to this challenge. When an AI system generates a recommendation, it can create the illusion of certainty, a probability score of 87% feels authoritative even when it should not be. Students must be taught to interrogate the basis of AI confidence claims, to understand the difference between a model's accuracy on a validation dataset and its reliability in a specific clinical context, and to maintain their own independent clinical reasoning as the primary framework, even when AI assistance is available.

17.7 Lifelong Learning: Building the Habit That Sustains a Career

A physician who believes their training ends at graduation has made a dangerous mistake. The knowledge they leave with will be partially obsolete within a decade. The AI tools they learn to use in training will be replaced by more advanced systems. The guidelines they follow will be updated by new evidence. New diseases and clinical challenges will continue to emerge. The patients they will serve will change in ways that cannot be predicted.

Lifelong learning is not optional; it is a professional obligation. And like every other professional competency, it must be taught, practiced, and assessed in medical school, not merely encouraged as a virtue.

World-class medical education builds lifelong learning as a habit, through regular personal learning plans that students develop and review; through research methodology training that enables students to read primary literature independently; through digital health literacy that ensures students can navigate the rapidly evolving landscape of AI tools and digital platforms; and through a culture of intellectual humility that treats not-knowing as the beginning of learning rather than a professional failure.

The Personal Learning System, What Every Graduate Must Be Able to Do
• Set personal learning goals: identify specific knowledge and skill gaps through self-assessment, feedback, and performance data, and set SMART goals to address them • Use quality learning resources: navigate primary literature, clinical guidelines, systematic reviews, and AI knowledge tools, critically evaluating the quality of each source • Schedule protected learning time: maintain a personal CPD calendar that treats learning as a non-negotiable professional obligation, not a residual activity • Seek and use feedback: actively request feedback from peers, supervisors, and patients, and use it to update practice rather than defend it • Participate in communities of practice: grand rounds, journal clubs, professional society meetings, online professional communities, learning with and from peers throughout a career • Document and reflect: maintain a professional portfolio that records learning experiences, reflections, and competency development, required by NMC, ACGME, and GMC continuing professional development frameworks

- Teach to learn: the most powerful learning strategy is teaching, explaining concepts to others reveals gaps and deepens understanding. Every physician should be a teacher throughout their career

★ KEY TAKEAWAYS

1. Building a physician requires shaping a complete person, not delivering a curriculum. The medical educator's responsibility is developmental, not informational.
2. World-class knowledge architecture has three layers: foundational science (understanding), core clinical knowledge (learned), and navigational knowledge (knowing where to find the rest).
3. The year-by-year competency framework, from foundational science through supervised independence, provides the developmental map that curriculum must be designed to support.
4. Clinical skills must be taught, practiced in simulation before patient contact, and maintained throughout training, with AI as enhancement, never as replacement for independent competency.
5. Communication is patient safety: the evidence that communication quality directly affects clinical outcomes is unambiguous and must drive curriculum priority decisions.
6. Decision-making under uncertainty must be explicitly taught, including how to critically interrogate AI confidence scores and maintain independent clinical reasoning alongside AI tools.
7. Lifelong learning is a professional obligation built as a habit in medical school, through personal learning systems, research literacy, and a culture of intellectual humility.

▶ COMING NEXT

Chapter 17A goes deeper into the heart of what this book stands for, the precise criteria that define a world-class doctor and a world-class human being. Soft skills, human values, leadership, and human-

centered thinking: what they are, how top global medical colleges teach them, and how every medical institution can do the same.

Chapter 17A

World-Class Criteria: The Best Doctors and the Best Humans

Soft Skills, Human Values, Leadership, and Human-Centered Thinking, The Criteria, The Teaching, and the Global Benchmarks

> *"Wherever the art of medicine is loved, there is also a love of humanity."*
>
> **Hippocrates, whose 2,500-year-old insight remains the most precise definition of what separates a world-class doctor from a merely competent one.**

17A.1 Introduction: The Missing Half of Medical Education

Every graduating medical student should be able to meet a test that cannot be measured through written examinations alone, not an OSCE station, not a research viva. It is both simpler and more demanding than any formal examination. It is this: can this doctor walk into a room where a frightened patient is sitting alone, and within five minutes, make that patient feel genuinely heard, genuinely respected, and genuinely confident that they are in good hands?

Clinical knowledge is necessary for that outcome. But it is not sufficient. What makes the difference is everything that medical education has historically treated as secondary, the soft skills, the human values, the emotional intelligence, the leadership presence, and the human-centered thinking that distinguish a world-class physician from a technically adequate one.

This chapter defines the criteria for a world-class physician with precision. It examines what the best medical colleges in the world, Johns Hopkins, Harvard Medical School, AIIMS Delhi, CMC Vellore, the Karolinska

Institute, and the University of Melbourne, are doing to develop these qualities systematically. And it provides a practical framework for how any medical college, including Bhagyoday, can build these capabilities into its curriculum, culture, and assessment systems.

The central argument of this chapter is straightforward and supported by decades of evidence: soft skills are not peripheral to medicine. They are central to it. These skills can be systematically taught and rigorously assessed. And the institutions that teach them well produce doctors who are genuinely better, for their patients, for their colleagues, for their communities, and for themselves.

17A.2 The World-Class Doctor Criteria: A Precise Framework

What exactly does world-class mean when applied to a physician? The answer is not vague; it is specific, measurable, and achievable through deliberate educational design. The world-class physician meets defined criteria across three domains: clinical mastery (addressed throughout this book), soft skills excellence, and human values formation. All three are equally non-negotiable.

The following framework defines the criteria for each domain, not as aspirations, but as observable, assessable standards that every medical college must build its curriculum around.

THE WORLD-CLASS PHYSICIAN CRITERIA

C

CRITERION 1, COMMUNICATION MASTERY

World-class physicians communicate with precision, clarity, and compassion in every clinical encounter, from the first introduction to a new patient, to the delivery of a devastating diagnosis, to the coordination of a complex handover. They adapt their language to the patient's literacy level, cultural context, and emotional state. They listen as much as they speak. They check understanding. They document accurately. They write referral letters that colleagues can actually use. Communication is not a skill they use occasionally; it is the medium through which all of their clinical excellence reaches the patient.

Assessed by: OSCE communication stations; standardized patient feedback scores; video-reviewed consultation analysis; patient satisfaction surveys; 360-degree peer and supervisor feedback

C

CRITERION 2, EMOTIONAL INTELLIGENCE (EQ)

The world-class physician knows themselves, their triggers, their biases, their emotional responses under pressure, and manages them with consistent professionalism. They read the emotional state of patients, families, and colleagues accurately and respond appropriately. They do not bring their frustrations into the consultation room. They do not dismiss patient anxiety as irrational. They do not respond to a colleague's distress with indifference. High EQ is not a personality trait. It is a learnable competency, developed through structured reflection, feedback, coaching, and deliberate practice.

Assessed by: Emotional intelligence psychometric tools (EQ-i, Mayer-Salovey-Caruso); structured reflection portfolio; patient and colleague feedback; observational assessment by trained supervisors

C

CRITERION 3, LEADERSHIP ABILITY

The world-class physician leads, in the consultation room (guiding the patient), in the clinical team (leading the ward round, the emergency code, the multidisciplinary meeting), in the institution (contributing to quality improvement, governance, and education), and in the community (advocating for the health of the population they serve). Leadership in medicine is not about hierarchy; it is about taking responsibility for outcomes and creating the conditions for others to do their best work. It includes the courage to speak up when something is wrong, the wisdom to know when to defer, and the skill to build teams that function better than the sum of their parts.

Assessed by: Leadership project evaluation; 360-degree feedback from team members; quality improvement project outcomes; institutional leadership role performance; structured leadership reflection portfolio

C

CRITERION 4, EMPATHY AND COMPASSION

Empathy, the ability to accurately understand another person's emotional experience, and compassion, the motivation to act to relieve suffering, are the moral engines of medicine. Research is unambiguous: empathic physicians have patients with better adherence, better outcomes, fewer complaints, and higher satisfaction. Compassion prevents physician burnout by reconnecting the clinician to the meaning of their work. Both can be taught, through narrative medicine, Balint groups, patient shadowing, community immersion, and the deliberate cultivation of attentive presence. Both must be assessed, because what is not assessed sends the message that it does not matter.

Assessed by: Consultation observation using validated empathy scales (CARE Measure, JSPE); patient satisfaction specifically measuring empathy; narrative portfolio entries; peer observation and feedback

C

CRITERION 5, ETHICAL INTEGRITY

The world-class physician does the right thing, when it is easy and when it is hard. When the right thing is to tell a patient a difficult truth. When the right thing is to report a colleague's unsafe practice. When the right thing is to advocate for a patient who cannot advocate for themselves. When the right thing is to say 'I don't know' rather than fabricate confidence. Ethical integrity in the AI era extends to the transparency of AI use in clinical decisions, the protection of patient data, and the commitment to equitable care regardless of a patient's background. It is not rule-following; it is character, formed through education, modelling, and the lived experience of moral decision-making.

Assessed by: Ethics case discussions with structured assessment; AETCOM portfolio; scenario-based professional dilemmas assessment; observation of professional behaviour; faculty and peer reports of professional conduct

C

CRITERION 6, CULTURAL SENSITIVITY AND HEALTH EQUITY

The world-class physician provides equally excellent care to every patient, regardless of their caste, class, gender, religion, language, sexual orientation, disability, or economic status. They understand that health outcomes are shaped by social determinants, and that the physician who ignores these determinants is not practising evidence-based medicine. In both India and the United States, health disparities are documented, consequential, and addressable. The culturally sensitive physician asks not just 'what disease does this patient have' but 'what conditions in this patient's life are making them sick', and addresses both.

Assessed by: Cross-cultural communication OSCE stations; community health project assessment; health equity case reflection portfolio; structured observation in diverse patient populations

C

CRITERION 7, HUMAN-CENTERED THINKING

Human-centered thinking, borrowed from design thinking and applied to medicine, means beginning every clinical problem by deeply understanding the patient's perspective, not just their physiology. It means asking: what matters most to this patient? What does this diagnosis mean to their life, their family, their work, their identity? What barriers will they face in following this treatment plan? And how can I design a management approach that actually works for this specific human being, not just for a hypothetical average patient? In the AI era, human-centered thinking is the distinctively human capability that algorithms cannot replicate, and that every physician must develop to the highest level.

Assessed by: Patient journey mapping exercises; patient-centered consultation assessment; shared decision-making OSCE stations; patient-reported outcome measures from student consultations

17A.3 How Soft Skills Are Actually Taught: The Pedagogical Methods That Work

Knowing what world-class looks like is not enough. The critical question is: how? How do you actually teach empathy to a second-year medical student who has been told their whole academic life that success means correct answers on written examinations? How do you develop leadership in someone who has never been given real responsibility? How do you build genuine compassion in an institutional culture that implicitly rewards clinical efficiency over emotional engagement?

The answer is: through deliberate, structured, assessed practice, the same approach that is used to develop clinical skills. Not through lectures about empathy. Not through optional workshops on communication. Through curriculum-embedded, faculty-modelled, formally assessed, continuously practiced soft skill development that treats human capabilities with the same seriousness as anatomy or pharmacology.

The following methods are evidence-based and in use at the world's best medical colleges. Each is described with the specific technique, the soft skill it develops, the evidence for its effectiveness, and how it is implemented in practice.

Method 1: Standardised Patient Encounters with Video Review

Standardised patients (SPs), trained actors who portray patients with specific conditions, histories, and emotional states, are the gold standard for teaching and assessing communication and interpersonal skills. The student conducts a consultation with the SP exactly as they would with a real patient. The consultation is video-recorded. Immediately afterward, the student, the SP, and a faculty observer review the video together, identifying specific moments where communication was effective, and specific moments where it missed the mark.

This method works because feedback is immediate, specific, and tied to observable behaviour. The student sees exactly what the patient saw, the moment they looked at their notes instead of at the patient's face; the moment they used jargon that the SP clearly did not understand; the moment they interrupted before the patient had finished their thought. Seeing it on video makes it undeniable and learnable.

Johns Hopkins Medical School, Harvard Medical School, and AIIMS Delhi, all use SP-based video feedback as a core communication skills teaching method. At AIIMS, the Clinical Skills Lab runs SP encounters from the first year, ensuring students practice fundamental communication skills before they set foot on a ward.

Method 2: Narrative Medicine

Narrative medicine, developed by Dr. Rita Charon at Columbia University College of Physicians and Surgeons, teaches physicians to recognize, absorb, interpret, and be moved by the stories of illness. It uses literature, creative writing, and careful close reading of patient narratives to develop the attentive listening and empathic imagination that clinical communication requires.

In practice, narrative medicine sessions involve students reading a short text: a poem by a patient with cancer, a passage from a memoir about chronic illness, a short story about a family's experience of a loved one's dementia, and then writing briefly in response: what did you notice? What surprised you? What did it make you feel? Then sharing in a facilitated small group discussion.

Columbia's Program in Narrative Medicine is the most developed in the world, with a Master's degree program and faculty embedded in clinical departments that run narrative medicine rounds alongside traditional ward rounds. University College London, the University of Toronto, and Kasturba Medical College (Manipal, India) have adopted narrative medicine programs. The evidence shows that students who participate in narrative medicine programs score significantly higher on empathy assessments and report greater ability to sustain compassion under the pressure of clinical work.

Method 3: Balint Groups

Balint groups, developed by psychoanalyst Michael Balint in the 1950s, are small groups of six to twelve medical students or physicians who meet regularly (typically fortnightly) to discuss difficult clinical cases, not the medical complexity of the case, but the emotional and relational complexity. How did this patient make you feel? What was happening in the room that you did not say out loud? How did your own feelings affect your clinical decisions?

The explicit goal of Balint groups is to develop the physician's emotional self-awareness, their ability to recognize and manage the emotional responses that arise in clinical work, rather than suppressing them or acting them out. Balint groups are a protected space in which the emotional reality of medicine can be named honestly, which makes physicians safer clinicians and more resilient human beings.

The Tavistock Clinic in London has the most developed Balint tradition. They are used systematically in GP training in the UK, the Netherlands, Germany, and France. In India, CMC Vellore and St. John's Medical College, Bangalore have introduced Balint group programs for postgraduate trainees. The evidence shows that Balint group participation reduces burnout, increases empathy scores, and improves the doctor-patient relationship in measurable ways.

Method 4: Community Immersion and Service Learning

No classroom exercise can develop the understanding of social determinants of health: poverty, housing, food security, caste, discrimination, that shapes the real-world health of patients. Only direct community experience can do this. Community immersion programs place medical students in the communities they will eventually serve, living with rural families, working in urban slums, accompanying community health workers on their rounds, sitting with patients in their homes rather than across a clinic desk.

CMC Vellore has the most celebrated community immersion program in Indian medical education, placing every student in rural community health postings where they provide primary care under supervision and live in the community. This experience is widely cited by CMC graduates as the most transformative of their medical education. AIIMS Rishikesh similarly embeds community health postings throughout the curriculum.

In the United States, Harvard Medical School's Primary Care Clerkship includes community health center rotations in underserved Boston neighborhoods. UCSF has a Social Justice and Health Equity curriculum that includes structured community engagement from the first year. The evidence consistently shows that community immersion increases students' commitment to primary care, underserved populations, and health equity advocacy throughout their careers.

Method 5: Leadership Development Laboratories

Leadership cannot be taught through lectures alone. It is developed through experience, through taking responsibility for a team, navigating a conflict, making a decision with incomplete information, failing and recovering, and receiving feedback from people who were affected by your leadership. Medical education has historically provided almost none of this experience before graduation.

Leadership development laboratories create structured opportunities for medical students to exercise leadership in progressively challenging contexts: leading a student quality improvement team; facilitating a peer learning group; managing a community health project with real deliverables; serving as a student representative in institutional governance; leading a simulation emergency as incident commander.

The University of Toronto's MD program has a formal leadership curriculum embedded across all four years, culminating in a leadership capstone project in the final year. Duke-NUS Medical School in Singapore integrates leadership development with systems science from the first year, producing graduates who are simultaneously clinical leaders and healthcare innovators. At Bhagyoday, every student completes a quality improvement project in Year 3 that they lead from problem identification through data collection to solution implementation, developing genuine leadership experience before graduation.

Method 6: Schwartz Rounds

Schwartz Rounds, developed by the Schwartz Center for Compassionate Healthcare in Boston, are monthly multidisciplinary forums in which healthcare staff share the human stories of clinical work: a case that stayed with them, a moment of connection with a patient, a situation that broke their heart or restored their faith. Physicians, nurses, social workers, and chaplains sit together and listen to each other's experiences of providing care.

For medical students who observe or participate in Schwartz Rounds, the impact is profound. They see that the emotional experiences they are having, the grief, the moral distress, the moments of connection, are universal across the healthcare team. They learn that naming these experiences is not a weakness but wisdom. And they develop the emotional vocabulary and reflective capacity that sustain compassionate practice across a career.

Schwartz Rounds are now held in over 600 healthcare organizations in the United States and United Kingdom. The Royal College of Physicians and the King's Fund in the UK have championed their spread across the NHS. In India, Apollo Hospitals and Narayana Health have introduced Schwartz-style compassion forums. The evidence shows that regular participation reduces burnout, increases compassion satisfaction, and improves team cohesion in measurable ways.

17A.4 World-Class Medical Colleges: What They Are Actually Doing

Theory becomes persuasive when it is grounded in the practice of institutions that have demonstrated results. The following profiles examine what the world's top medical colleges are doing specifically to develop soft skills, human values, leadership, and human-centered thinking, and what lessons every institution can take from their experience.

Institution	Signature Soft Skill Program	What Makes It World-Class	Lesson for Every College
Johns Hopkins, USA	Genes to Society curriculum, longitudinal integration of social, psychological, and biological determinants; SP-based communication training from Week 1; required community health project	Treats social determinants as core medical science; SP communication training is not an add-on, it begins before first clinical contact; every student has a community health experience that connects medicine to real lives	Start communication skills training before clinical rotations. Make community health a required curriculum component, not an elective. Integrate social determinants into every clinical teaching case
Harvard Medical, USA	Doctoring course, longitudinal across all years; Schwartz Rounds; Patient-Doctor III focuses exclusively on communication in complex situations; primary care community health center rotations	Doctoring is treated as a distinct and equal discipline alongside basic science and clinical medicine; Schwartz Rounds are institution-wide, not just for students; community rotations are mandatory for all students	Dedicate curriculum time equal to other major subjects for human skills development. Run Schwartz Rounds or equivalent compassion forums as a permanent institutional practice
UCSF Medical, USA	Bridges Curriculum, collaborative learning, health equity longitudinal thread, reflective	Health equity is not a lecture; it is a longitudinal thread woven through every year. Student-run	Build a health equity thread across all years. Give students real clinical responsibility in

	writing from Year 1; Difference, Power and Discrimination module; student-run health clinics in underserved communities	clinics give real responsibility for underserved patient care. Reflective writing is formally assessed, not optional	underserved contexts. Formally assess reflective writing, make it count
Columbia University, USA	Program in Narrative Medicine, founded by Dr. Rita Charon; close reading and creative writing seminars; narrative medicine rounds in clinical departments; narrative competency assessed throughout	Narrative medicine is not an enrichment add-on; it has its own faculty, its own curriculum thread, and its own assessment. Clinical faculty run narrative medicine alongside ward rounds. Graduates publish narrative medicine research	Create a narrative medicine program with dedicated faculty. Embed narrative medicine in clinical departments, not just as a pre-clinical exercise but as a continuous clinical practice
Karolinska Institute, Sweden	Problem-Based Learning with interprofessional teams; mandatory global health rotations; ethics longitudinal thread; student research projects on health equity; peer teaching and assessment program	PBL teams are interprofessional, medicine, nursing, pharmacy, social work, developing teamwork skills from day one. Global health rotations develop cultural competency through genuine cross-cultural experience	Make interprofessional education mandatory from the first year. Give students global or cross-cultural clinical experiences. Require peer teaching, it develops communication and leadership simultaneously
CMC Vellore, India	Rural community health postings for all students; chapel services and spiritual care integration; pastoral care training; servant leadership model embedded in institutional culture; patient shadowing program	The institutional culture is itself the curriculum, values of service, humility, and compassion are lived by the faculty and absorbed by students. Rural postings are comprehensive, supervised, and reflective. Patient	Institutional culture matters more than curriculum documents. Faculty must live the values they are trying to teach. Patient shadowing, following a patient through their entire hospital journey, is

		shadowing builds genuine empathy	transformative and low-cost
AIIMS Delhi, India	Clinical Skills Lab with SP encounters from Year 1; AETCOM program for attitudes, ethics, and communication; interdepartmental case conferences with humanities integration; research from Year 2	AIIMS has made AETCOM genuinely rigorous; it is assessed, and assessment results are taken seriously. The Clinical Skills Lab is used from the very beginning of medical education. Research develops critical thinking from early in training	Implement AETCOM with genuine rigor, assess it and count the results. Give students clinical skills lab access from the first weeks of medical school. Begin supervised research from Year 2
University of Melbourne, Australia	Melbourne Curriculum, graduate-entry model; health humanities thread; clinical communication assessed at every year; Indigenous health and cultural safety mandatory module; interprofessional practice from Year 1	Graduate entry means students bring maturity and diverse life experience to medicine. Indigenous health and cultural safety is mandatory, not optional, and assessed. Communication is assessed at every year level, not just at graduation	Require cultural safety training as mandatory and assessed. Assess communication formally at every year of training. Value diverse prior experience in student selection, it enriches the cohort and develops human skills

17A.5 Human-Centered Thinking: Designing Medicine Around the Patient

Human-centered thinking, or human-centered design applied to medicine, is the practice of beginning every clinical and systems problem by deeply understanding the human being at its center. Not just their diagnosis. Not just their test results. Their life. Their fears. Their resources. Their relationships. Their definition of a good outcome.

This approach is not new to medicine in principle, patient-centered care has been a stated value for decades. What is new is the systematic application of design thinking methodology to medical education and practice: structured empathy research, patient journey mapping, co-design of care plans with patients, and iterative improvement of care processes based on patient experience data.

The Design Thinking Framework Applied to Medicine

Design thinking has five stages that are Empathize, Define, Ideate, Prototype, Test, that translate directly into a clinical problem-solving approach that puts the patient's experience at the center of every decision:

Stage	Design Thinking	Applied to Clinical Care	Teaching Method
1	**Empathize** Before forming a clinical impression, deeply understand the patient's experience, what their illness means to their life, family, work, and identity. Ask open questions. Listen without interrupting. Shadow patients through their healthcare journey.	Before forming a clinical impression, deeply understand the patient's experience, what their illness means to their life, family, work, and identity. Ask open questions. Listen without interrupting. Shadow patients through their healthcare journey.	Patient shadowing exercises; illness narrative writing from patient perspective; structured empathy interviews with real patients; trained SP encounters focused on deep listening rather than history structure
2	**Define** Frame the problem from the patient's perspective, not just the physician's. Not 'patient with poorly controlled diabetes' but 'a 58-year-old farmer who cannot afford insulin and has no transport to the clinic', the real problem includes the social context.	Frame the problem from the patient's perspective, not just the physician's. Not 'patient with poorly controlled diabetes' but 'a 58-year-old farmer who cannot afford insulin and has no transport to the clinic', the real problem includes the social context.	Patient journey mapping workshops; social determinants screening tools; community health field visits; interprofessional team case formulation exercises that include patient-defined problems
3	**Ideate** Generate multiple possible approaches to the patient's problem, including non-medical approaches that	Generate multiple possible approaches to the patient's problem, including non-medical approaches that	Multidisciplinary case conferences with patient and family participation; shared decision-making training; patient decision aid co-design workshops;

	address social determinants, patient-reported barriers, and patient preferences. Avoid anchoring on the first solution.	address social determinants, patient-reported barriers, and patient preferences. Avoid anchoring on the first solution.	creative problem-solving seminars with real cases
4	**Prototype** Develop a management plan collaboratively with the patient, not for the patient. Test the plan against the patient's actual life: Can they afford this? Can they take time off work for this appointment? Does this fit with their cultural or religious values?	Develop a management plan collaboratively with the patient, not for the patient. Test the plan against the patient's actual life: Can they afford this? Can they take time off work for this appointment? Does this fit with their cultural or religious values?	Motivational interviewing training; health literacy assessment and communication adaptation; patient teach-back technique practice; culturally adapted care planning exercises
5	**Test** Follow up to see whether the plan worked, not just clinically, but from the patient's perspective. Collect patient-reported outcomes. Ask what worked and what did not. Revise based on what you learn. Improvement is continuous.	Follow up to see whether the plan worked, not just clinically, but from the patient's perspective. Collect patient-reported outcomes. Ask what worked and what did not. Revise based on what you learn. Improvement is continuous.	Patient-reported outcome measurement training; follow-up consultation skills; shared care plan review techniques; quality improvement methodology applied to individual patient management

17A.6 How Soft Skills Are Assessed: Making the Invisible Measurable

The single most important institutional signal about what matters is what is formally assessed. When soft skills are taught but not assessed, or assessed but the results are not taken seriously, students receive a clear message: these things matter less than the scores that actually count.

World-class institutions close this gap by assessing soft skills with the same rigour they apply to clinical knowledge.

The Soft Skill Assessment Portfolio, Tools Every Medical College Must Implement

- 360-Degree Feedback: structured feedback from patients, peers, nurses, allied health staff, and supervisors, covering communication, empathy, professionalism, and teamwork. Minimum twice per year from Year 3 onward. Results reviewed in faculty mentoring sessions with personalised development planning
- OSCE Communication Stations: dedicated OSCE stations assessing specific communication competencies, history-taking empathy, breaking bad news, shared decision-making, cross-cultural communication, telephone consultation, discharge planning. Each station scored by trained assessors using validated rubrics. Minimum 30% of the total OSCE score
- Mini-CEX (Mini Clinical Evaluation Exercise): brief structured observations of real clinical encounters by supervising faculty, 15-20 minutes of observation followed by immediate feedback. Assessed on history, physical examination, communication, clinical judgement, professionalism, and organisation. Minimum 6 per year in clinical years
- Narrative Portfolio with Structured Reflection: written reflections on clinical encounters, ethical dilemmas, leadership experiences, and community health observations, assessed against a reflective depth framework (description → analysis → synthesis → transformation). Required for progression at each year level
- Patient Satisfaction Surveys: structured patient feedback on specific student consultations, measuring respect, listening, explanation clarity, and whether the patient felt genuinely cared for. Aggregated anonymously and shared with students quarterly as learning data
- Leadership Project Assessment: formal evaluation of the student's quality improvement or community health leadership project, assessed on problem definition, team leadership, stakeholder engagement, data use, implementation, and results. Weighted as a major assessment component in Years 3-4

- Peer Assessment: structured peer feedback on communication, teamwork, and professional behaviour in small group and clinical team settings. Anonymised, aggregated, and reviewed with faculty mentor. Develops the habit of seeking and giving feedback that sustains professional development throughout a career

★ KEY TAKEAWAYS

8. World-class doctors are defined by seven precise criteria: Communication Mastery, Emotional Intelligence, Leadership Ability, Empathy and Compassion, Ethical Integrity, Cultural Sensitivity, and Human-Centered Thinking, all measurable and all teachable.
9. Soft skills are not peripheral to medicine; they are central to it. The evidence that communication, empathy, and human values directly improve patient outcomes is unambiguous and decades-deep.
10. Six evidence-based teaching methods develop soft skills systematically: SP encounters with video feedback, narrative medicine, Balint groups, community immersion, leadership laboratories, and Schwartz Rounds.
11. Johns Hopkins, Harvard, UCSF, Columbia, Karolinska, CMC Vellore, AIIMS Delhi, and the University of Melbourne are the global benchmarks, each with a signature approach that every college can learn from and adapt.
12. Human-centered thinking, the five-stage design thinking framework applied to medicine, puts the patient's full lived experience at the center of every clinical problem and every care plan.
13. Soft skills must be formally assessed: 360-degree feedback, OSCE communication stations, Mini-CEX, narrative portfolio, patient satisfaction surveys, leadership project evaluation, and peer assessment.
14. The measure of a world-class medical college is simple: do its graduates make every patient feel genuinely heard, genuinely respected, and genuinely cared for, consistently, across every kind of encounter?

▶ COMING NEXT

Chapter 18, the final chapter of Part 5, focuses on the faculty: the teachers, mentors, and role models who make or break every educational program. How do we develop faculty who can teach with passion, integrate AI into their practice and teaching, and lead the transformation of medical education from the inside?

Chapter 18

Faculty Development for Excellence

Training Faculty in AI, Teaching With Passion, Mentorship, and Leading Educational Transformation

> *"The mediocre teacher tells. The good teacher explains. The superior teacher demonstrates. The great teacher inspires."*
>
> **William Arthur Ward, the standard against which every medical educator must measure their impact on the physicians they are shaping.**

18.1 Introduction: Faculty Are the Curriculum

There is a saying in medical education that is as true today as it has ever been: the hidden curriculum is more powerful than the formal curriculum. What students actually learn, the values they internalize, the professional habits they form, the model of medicine they carry into their careers, comes primarily not from what is written in the curriculum document, but from what they observe in the faculty who teach, supervise, and mentor them.

A faculty member who treats nurses dismissively teaches students that nursing colleagues are subordinate rather than partners. One who documents meticulously teaches the value of clinical records One who says, “I don’t know. Let’s look it up together,” models the intellectual humility that sustains lifelong learning. One who uses AI tools critically and explains their reasoning aloud teaches AI literacy more effectively than any lecture.

Faculty are the curriculum. Every other investment in medical education, simulation centres, AI platforms, library resources, curriculum redesign, is multiplied or undermined by the quality of the people who stand in front of students, supervise their clinical work, and shape their professional identity.

This chapter addresses the most important and most frequently neglected dimension of medical education improvement: the development of faculty. It examines what exceptional medical faculty do, how AI is changing the faculty role, how to build faculty AI literacy, and what a world-class faculty development program looks like for institutions like Bhagyoday.

18.2 What Exceptional Medical Faculty Do: The Evidence

Research on effective medical teaching, from the CanMEDS Scholar role to ACGME faculty development standards, identifies consistent characteristics of faculty who produce exceptional learning outcomes in their students. These characteristics are not personality traits that people either possess or lack. They are learnable competencies that faculty development programs can build.

L1	**Foundational Teaching Competency, Every Faculty Member** **Who:** All teaching faculty, clinical and non-clinical, within the first year of appointment **What:** Structured teaching skills (how to plan and deliver a teaching session); effective feedback techniques (SMART feedback, not vague praise such as "good job"); basic adult learning principles; patient communication modelling; CBME competency framework orientation; AI literacy foundation; NMC teaching obligations and documentation **Outcome:** *Faculty can plan coherent learning sessions, deliver structured feedback, and model evidence-based clinical practice. Meets NMC minimum faculty qualification requirements.*
L2	**Advanced Teaching Excellence, Senior Faculty and Department Leads** **Who:** Faculty with 3+ years teaching experience; all department heads; clinical supervisors for the final year and internship **What:** Small group facilitation for PBL and TBL; simulation-based teaching design and facilitation; OSCE station design and examiner training; curriculum mapping and learning outcome design; student assessment and portfolio

	review; AI in clinical teaching, how to supervise AI tool use in clinical settings; quality improvement in teaching, how to measure and improve your own teaching **Outcome:** *Faculty can design curriculum components, lead small group learning, design and run OSCE assessments, and supervise student AI use in clinical practice.*
L3	**Educational Leadership, Curriculum Leaders and Academic Heads** **Who:** Heads of departments; curriculum committee members; programme directors; assessment committee leads **What:** Curriculum design at programme level; competency framework development; NMC CBME implementation leadership; faculty development programme design; educational research methodology; AI curriculum integration strategy; NABH + NMC dual accreditation alignment; educational quality management and accreditation preparation **Outcome:** *Faculty can lead curriculum transformation, design faculty development programmes, manage accreditation processes, and drive institution-wide educational quality improvement.*
L4	**Medical Education Scholar, Research and National Leadership** **Who:** Selected faculty with educational research interests and institutional leadership aspirations **What:** Postgraduate medical education qualification (PGCert/MEd/PhD in Medical Education); educational research design and publication; national curriculum development participation; conference presentation and knowledge dissemination; mentorship of junior faculty educators; AI in medical education research, contribution to the evidence base **Outcome:** *Faculty who advance the field of medical education nationally and internationally, contributing research, shaping policy, and developing the next generation of medical educators.*

18.3 Training Faculty in AI: Building the Teaching Team of the Future

For faculty development in AI, three distinct but related competencies must be built: AI as a clinical tool (how to use and critically evaluate AI in their own clinical practice), AI as a teaching tool (how to integrate AI into their teaching effectively), and AI as a subject to teach (how to develop students' own AI literacy and critical evaluation skills).

These are not the same competency. A faculty member may be comfortable using an AI diagnostic tool in their clinical work but uncertain about how to create a learning experience that develops students' critical AI evaluation skills. A faculty member may understand the AI literacy conceptually but not know how to facilitate a case conference in which AI tool outputs are interrogated as part of the clinical reasoning process.

Faculty development in AI must address all three levels and must be updated regularly, because the AI landscape in healthcare and education is evolving faster than any other technology in the history of the profession.

Faculty AI Development Programme, Core Content at Each Level

- FOUNDATION (all faculty): What AI is and how it works; FDA/CDSCO cleared tools in your specialty; how to evaluate AI recommendations critically; HIPAA/GDPR and patient data privacy with AI tools; AI ethics principles and patient disclosure; AI learning tools available to students, how they work and how to support effective use
- INTERMEDIATE (senior faculty): AI performance metrics, sensitivity, specificity, PPV, NPV, and how to interpret them clinically; bias in AI and how to identify it; how to supervise students using AI in clinical settings; designing AI-integrated teaching sessions and assessments; AI in research, literature review, manuscript assistance, data analysis support
- ADVANCED (department heads and curriculum leads): AI governance and ethics committee participation; AI curriculum integration strategy at department level; AI implementation leadership, faculty champion role in hospital AI deployments; evaluating AI vendors for educational and clinical use; AI educational research, contributing to the evidence base on AI in medical education

- ONGOING (all levels): Quarterly AI update sessions, new tools, new evidence, new regulatory developments; peer observation of AI-integrated teaching with structured feedback; case discussions on AI performance issues encountered in clinical or teaching settings; annual AI literacy self-assessment and personal development planning

18.4 Teaching With Passion: The Human Dimension of Faculty Excellence

All the technology, curriculum design, and competency frameworks in this chapter will fail if the faculty members deploying them do not bring genuine passion to their teaching. Passion in education is not performance; it is not enthusiasm manufactured for the classroom. It is the authentic expression of a faculty member who is genuinely excited by their subject, genuinely invested in their students' development, and genuinely committed to the mission of producing excellent physicians.

Passion is contagious. A faculty member who loves biochemistry and communicates that passion, showing students why metabolic pathways are intellectually beautiful as well as clinically important, produces students who engage with the subject very differently from those taught by someone delivering the same material as a compliance exercise.

Passion is also sustaining. Medical faculty carry enormous workloads, clinical service, teaching, research, administration, and the ongoing development of their own expertise. Without a genuine sense of purpose and love for the work, burnout is almost inevitable. Faculty development programs that address not just competencies but meaning, why this work matters, what difference excellent teaching makes, what it feels like to watch a student become a physician, sustain the passion that sustains the teaching.

At Bhagyoday, faculty development includes explicit attention to the question of purpose: Why do you teach? What do you want your students to remember about you in 20 years? What difference will you make to the physicians you are developing, and through them, to the patients they will serve? These are not soft questions peripheral to the curriculum. They are the questions that determine whether faculty development produces teachers or inspires educators.

18.5 Mentorship and Leadership: The Faculty's Most Enduring Impact

Teaching delivers knowledge. Mentorship shapes identity. The distinction is important, because it is the mentor who a physician remembers and models across their career, far more than the content of any particular lecture or examination.

Great mentors in medicine do specific things: they know their mentees as individuals: their strengths, doubts, and aspirations; they create the psychological safety that allows mentees to be honest about their struggles; they offer honest feedback delivered with genuine care; they open doors, to clinical opportunities, to research collaborations, to professional networks, that mentees could not open alone; and they model the complete physician identity that the mentee is working toward, in their own clinical practice, their own learning habits, and their own human relationships.

Every Bhagyoday student has a designated faculty mentor from the first week of the program to the final day of internship. Mentoring relationships are not optional, not informal, and not based on chance encounters in the corridor. They are structured, scheduled, documented, and supported by training for faculty in the specific skills of effective mentorship.

What Great Mentors Do	What Poor Mentorship Looks Like
Know the mentee as an individual, their goals, struggles, and context	Treat all mentees identically, one-size-fits-all advice and support
Create psychological safety, honest conversations without judgment	Create fear, mentees hide struggles rather than risk being seen as weak
Give specific, actionable, honest feedback, with genuine care	Give vague praise or harsh criticism, neither of which enables growth
Open professional doors: introductions, opportunities, advocacy	Operate as a gatekeeper, take credit for student work, and create barriers to opportunity
Model intellectual humility, 'I don't know, let's find out together'	Project false certainty; never admits a gap in knowledge or a mistake
Celebrate student achievements genuinely and publicly	Take credit for student successes while assigning blame for failures
Maintain appropriate boundaries while being genuinely invested	Either distant and transactional or inappropriately close and dependent
Review and adjust the mentoring relationship as the student develops	Maintain the same relationship pattern regardless of student progress

18.6 Faculty Wellbeing: The Foundation of Sustainable Excellence

Faculty cannot give what they do not have. A burned-out, chronically stressed, inadequately supported faculty member cannot inspire students, deliver excellent teaching, or model the professional well-being that students need to see embodied in the physicians they are becoming.

Faculty well-being is not a peripheral concern; it is a strategic imperative for medical education quality. Research consistently shows that faculty burnout directly impairs teaching quality, reduces engagement with students, increases cynicism in the hidden curriculum, and, most damagingly, models exactly the professional deterioration that medical education should be protecting against.

World-class institutions invest in faculty wellbeing with the same seriousness they invest in student wellbeing: protected time for scholarly activities and personal development; manageable teaching and clinical service ratios; recognition and reward systems that value teaching excellence alongside research productivity; peer support networks; and institutional cultures that model the humane, sustainable professional life that medical students should aspire to, not just in their patients' lives but in their own

★ KEY TAKEAWAYS

15. Faculty are the curriculum, the hidden curriculum conveyed through faculty behaviour and values shapes physicians more powerfully than any formal curriculum document.
16. Exceptional medical faculty demonstrate specific learnable competencies: inspiring teaching, structured feedback, intellectual humility, mentorship, and modelling of professional values.
17. The Faculty Development Ladder, Foundation, Advanced, Educational Leadership and Scholar, provides a structured progression framework for building a world-class teaching team.
18. AI faculty development requires three distinct competencies: AI as clinical tool, AI as teaching tool, and AI as a subject to teach, updated quarterly as the technology evolves.
19. Teaching with passion is not performance; it is the authentic expression of faculty who love their subject and their students. Passion is contagious and sustaining and must be protected.
20. Mentorship shapes professional identity more powerfully than teaching delivers content, every student deserves a designated, trained, genuinely invested faculty mentor.
21. Faculty wellbeing is a strategic imperative: burned-out faculty cannot inspire students, model professional flourishing, or sustain the teaching excellence that student outcomes require.
22. The Bhagyoday faculty model, recruited for values, trained before student contact, developed continuously, recognised for teaching, is the blueprint for building a world-class teaching institution.

▶ COMING NEXT

Part 6 turns from vision and education to implementation, the practical journey of converting these principles into reality. Chapter 19 provides the AI Implementation Roadmap: the step-by-step framework from awareness through training, pilot, and scale. This is where strategy meets action.

PART SIX

Implementation, From Vision to Reality

The practical frameworks, change leadership tools, and real-world case study that turn strategy into action

Chapter 19

AI Implementation Roadmap

Awareness → Training → Pilot → Scale, A Step-by-Step Framework for Every Hospital

> *"Vision without execution is hallucination."*
>
> **Thomas Edison whose laboratories produced not just ideas but working systems. The same discipline separates AI vision from AI impact in healthcare.**

19.1 Introduction: Why Most AI Implementations Fail, and How Yours Will Succeed

The global healthcare AI market is projected to exceed $150 billion by 2030. Hospitals around the world are investing in AI diagnostic tools, clinical decision support systems, operational optimization platforms, and AI-powered medical education. And yet, the majority of AI implementations in healthcare fail to deliver their promised value. Not because the technology does not work. Because the implementation does.

Studies of healthcare AI adoption consistently identify the same pattern of failure: a technology-first approach that purchases a sophisticated AI system without first ensuring the data quality, workflow integration, staff training, governance structure, and cultural readiness that make AI work in practice. The AI is deployed. Clinicians do not trust it. Alert fatigue sets in. The system is bypassed. The investment is written off. Leadership moves to the next technology trend.

This chapter provides a different approach, a structured, four-phase implementation roadmap that begins with awareness, progresses through training, moves carefully through piloting, and only then scales. Each phase has defined entry and exit criteria, specific actions, measurable success metrics, and risk mitigation strategies. This is not a theoretical framework. It is grounded in the quality management principles, change leadership practices, and AI governance requirements established throughout this book, and it is the framework being applied at Bhagyoday Hospital.

19.2 Pre-Implementation: The Readiness Assessment

Before any implementation phase begins, every hospital must conduct an honest readiness assessment. This is not a vendor demonstration. It is a structured internal audit of the organisation's current capability across six dimensions. The readiness assessment determines which AI applications are appropriate given current maturity, what foundational work must be completed before implementation, and what realistic timelines look like.

Readiness Dimension	Ready (Score 3)	Partial (Score 2)	Not Ready (Score 1)
Data Infrastructure	Comprehensive EHR with clean, structured data; FHIR-compliant APIs; automated data flows from all clinical devices	EHR implemented, but data quality issues; some manual data entry; partial device integration	Paper-based or minimal EHR; significant data gaps; no device integration; data quality unknown
IT Infrastructure	Stable network across all departments; adequate computing resources; dedicated IT staff for healthcare systems	Network coverage patchy; limited IT staff; computing resources constrained	Minimal IT infrastructure; no dedicated healthcare IT staff; network unreliable
Leadership Commitment	CEO/CMO explicitly championing AI; board-level AI governance; AI strategy formally	Leadership supportive but not visibly leading; no formal governance; AI in strategy	No explicit leadership position on AI; viewed as IT project; no governance or budget allocated

	approved and resourced	documents but not budgeted	
Staff Readiness	Foundational AI literacy training completed across all departments; champions identified in clinical areas	Awareness workshops held for some staff; champions not yet formally identified	No AI literacy training; staff unaware or anxious about AI; no champions
Quality & Safety Systems	Robust quality management system; incident reporting culture; performance measurement in place	Basic quality systems; some safety reporting; measurement ad hoc	No formal quality system; blame culture; minimal measurement
Governance & Ethics	AI Ethics Committee established; AI governance policy approved; bias auditing protocol defined	AI governance being developed; policy in draft; committee not yet formed	No AI governance; no ethics committee; no policy for AI deployment

Score each dimension 1–3 and total. Scores of 15–18: The organization is ready to begin Phase 1.Scores of 10–14: complete the Not Ready items before beginning; expect 6–12 months of foundational work. Scores below 10: significant foundational investment required before any AI implementation; focus first on EHR, data quality, and leadership alignment. Attempting to deploy AI with a score below 10 is the single most common cause of failed healthcare AI implementations.

19.3 The Four-Phase Implementation Roadmap

The roadmap that follows is not prescriptive in timeline; it is prescriptive in sequence. Every phase must be substantially completed before the next begins. Shortcuts produce the failed implementations described in the introduction. Discipline in the sequence produces the sustainable results that justify AI investment and build the organisational confidence for continued expansion.

Phase 1, AWARENESS | *Months 1–6* *Goal: Build organisation-wide understanding of AI, what it is, what it can do, what it requires, and how it will be governed*		
Key Actions	**Success Metrics**	**Key Risks & Mitigations**
• AI literacy workshops for all staff, role-specific content (clinicians, nurses, administrators, board) • Senior leadership AI education, board briefings, CMO/CEO strategic AI workshop • Current state assessment, data quality audit, workflow mapping, vendor landscape review • AI Ethics Committee formation, recruit members, draft charter, establish meeting cadence • AI strategy development, identify 3 priority use cases aligned to strategic goals • Vendor landscape analysis, evaluate AI tools available for priority use cases • Patient and community	• 100% of clinical staff completed AI awareness training • AI Ethics Committee convened with all required roles represented • 3 priority AI use cases formally approved by leadership • Baseline KPIs documented for all priority areas • Data quality assessment completed with improvement plan • AI governance policy in draft for committee review	• Risk: Leadership enthusiasm wanes before action, Mitigation: Assign AI champion at C-suite level with explicit accountability • Risk: Training felt as burden not opportunity, Mitigation: Make training relevant to each role; use real local clinical examples • Risk: Vendor pressure to skip to deployment, Mitigation: No vendor contracts until Phase 2 criteria are met

communication, develop AI transparency statement for public • Baseline measurement, document current performance on KPIs AI will target		

Phase 2, TRAINING | *Months 4–12 (overlaps Phase 1 exit)*

Goal: Develop deep competency in the specific AI systems selected, and complete the data and governance foundations required for safe deployment

Key Actions	Success Metrics	Key Risks & Mitigations
• Vendor selection, formal RFP, clinical evaluation, reference site visits, contract negotiation including BAA/GDPR/data agreements • Local validation study, test AI performance on your patient population BEFORE clinical deployment • Deep-dive training, system-specific training for all users, including hands-on practice with realistic scenarios	• Local validation study completed with satisfactory performance metrics • All pilot-site staff completed system-specific training (>95% completion) • AI Ethics Committee has formally approved deployment for pilot • Downtime procedures	• Risk: Local validation shows poor performance, Mitigation: This indicates that the validation process is working correctly. Do not deploy; return to vendor for recalibration or select alternative • Risk: Training not retained without practice, Mitigation: Schedule go-live within 2 weeks of training completion; provide champion support at go-live • Risk: Integration failures discovered

• Downtime procedure development, documented workflows for when AI system is unavailable • Integration testing, validate data flows between EHR, devices, and AI systems • AI Ethics Committee review, formal pre-deployment review of evidence, governance plan, bias audit • Clinical champion training, intensive preparation of department AI champions who will support colleagues • Communication campaign, prepare clinical teams for upcoming pilot; address concerns proactively	documented and tested • EHR and device integration tested and verified • Clinical champion team in place in each pilot department	late, Mitigation: Test in staging environment for minimum 4 weeks before go-live

Phase 3, PILOT | *Months 10–18 (overlaps Training exit)*

Goal: Deploy AI in a defined, monitored pilot environment, generating real performance data while protecting the broader organisation from unvalidated risk

Key Actions	**Success Metrics**	**Key Risks & Mitigations**
• Pilot site go-live, one department or ward; full support from champions and IT • Daily monitoring, performance dashboard reviewed daily for first 4 weeks • Weekly learning huddles, pilot team meets weekly to share experience and resolve issues • Alert calibration, adjust thresholds based on real clinical feedback; reduce alert fatigue • Outcome data collection, track pilot KPIs daily; compare to pre-implementation baseline • Bias audit, first formal audit of AI performance across demographic subgroups in pilot population	• AI system sensitivity and specificity within 10% of validation study in real-world use • Alert fatigue rate <20% (>80% of alerts reviewed by clinicians within required timeframe) • No AI-related adverse events or near-misses during pilot period • Pilot KPIs showing direction of improvement vs. baseline • Clinician satisfaction with AI tool >70% in structured survey • Bias audit shows no significant performance disparity across	• Risk: Clinical team bypasses AI system, Mitigation: Understand root cause; involve clinical champions in workflow redesign; do not force adoption • Risk: KPIs not improving, Mitigation: Return to DMAIC analysis; identify whether issue is data, algorithm, workflow, or training • Risk: Bias detected in pilot population, Mitigation: Suspend deployment; work with vendor on recalibration; re-audit before expansion

• Incident tracking, all AI-related concerns documented and reviewed by Ethics Committee • Expansion planning, based on pilot data, define criteria and timeline for Phase 4	demographic groups	

Phase 4, SCALE | *Months 16–36 (begins when pilot criteria fully met)*

Goal: Expand validated AI systems across the organisation, systematically, with sustained governance, and with continuous improvement embedded in operations

Key Actions	Success Metrics	Key Risks & Mitigations
• Phased departmental rollout, one department per month with dedicated champion and support • Peer learning network, pilot site champions mentor expansion site champions • Performance dashboard expansion, all sites reporting to unified quality dashboard	• All target departments live within planned timeline • Organisation-wide AI KPIs showing sustained improvement vs. pre-implementation baseline • Monthly Ethics Committee reviews completed with documented outcomes • Zero AI-related serious adverse events	• Risk: Expansion outpaces governance capacity, Mitigation: Governance committee size and meeting frequency scales with number of live systems • Risk: Performance drift detected, Mitigation: Drift monitoring protocol triggers automatic review and retraining process

• Quarterly AI governance review, Ethics Committee reviews all live systems; performance, bias, incidents • Model drift monitoring, establish protocol for detecting when AI model performance degrades over time • New use case evaluation, apply Phase 1–3 process to next priority AI applications • Staff refresher training, annual re-certification on all live AI systems • Public reporting, annual AI governance report published for patients and community	• Staff AI satisfaction score >80% organisation-wide • Annual bias audit completed across all demographic groups for all live systems	• Risk: Staff fatigue with training requirements, Mitigation: Annual refresher made efficient and relevant; champions deliver peer training rather than external programs

19.4 AI Use Case Prioritisation: Where to Start

With four phases clear, the practical question is: which AI application should a hospital implement first? The answer depends on the hospital's readiness profile, strategic priorities, and available resources, but the following framework guides the selection decision for any hospital, in any context, in both USA and India.

Start Here, High Impact, Lower Complexity	Build To, Moderate Complexity, High Value	Plan For: Complex, Transformative
• Sepsis early warning: high evidence base, clear clinical pathway, significant mortality impact, available as EHR-integrated tools • AI radiology: chest X-ray AI for TB screening (India) or pneumonia detection; FDA/CDSCO cleared tools available; radiologist-friendly workflow • Medication error reduction:	• AI clinical documentation: reduces physician documentation burden by 40-60%; improves data quality for downstream AI; requires EHR integration and clinical validation • Predictive readmission: requires 12+ months of clean historical data; clear care coordination workflow; significant financial and quality impact • ICU deterioration prediction: high	• AI-integrated surgical planning: high complexity; requires imaging AI, surgical team training, and outcome tracking infrastructure • Genomic medicine AI: precision oncology and pharmacogenomics; requires genomics lab infrastructure and specialist interpretation • AI for drug discovery and clinical trials: research-grade infrastructure; partnership with academic institutions required • Fully integrated patient journey AI: requires unified data platform across all

barcode administration AI and drug interaction checking; strong safety case; staff-appreciated reduction in error risk • Appointment scheduling optimisation: administrative AI with clear ROI; no clinical risk; builds AI confidence across non-clinical staff • Patient fall prediction: strong evidence, clear nursing workflow integration, immediate patient safety benefit	acuity environment requires rigorous validation; significant mortality benefit; requires device integration • AI-powered diagnostic pathways: cardiology, oncology, neurology, specialist-specific tools with strong evidence; requires specialty champion ownership • Population health management: requires ABDM/EHR data at scale; high community health impact; requires public health partnership	departments; Phase 4 maturity minimum • AI medical education platform: simulation, personalised learning, OSCE AI, requires medical college infrastructure and faculty development

19.5 The Vendor Selection Framework: Buying AI Responsibly

AI vendor selection is one of the highest-stakes procurement decisions a healthcare organisation makes, because AI vendors are not just software suppliers. They are partners in patient care, data custodians, and governance co-participants. The following criteria must govern every AI vendor selection process, regardless of price pressure or relationship history.

AI Vendor Evaluation Criteria, The Non-Negotiables

- Clinical evidence: peer-reviewed validation studies on populations similar to yours, not just developer-produced white papers. Sensitivity, specificity, PPV, and NPV reported separately for relevant demographic subgroups
- Regulatory status: FDA clearance (USA), CDSCO registration (India), CE Marking (EU-facing), verify independently, not from vendor claims
- Data privacy compliance: HIPAA Business Associate Agreement (USA), GDPR Standard Contractual Clauses (EU patients), DPDPA compliance (India), executed before any patient data is shared
- Interoperability: HL7 FHIR R4 API support verified by your technical team, not vendor claims. Test with your EHR in your environment
- Explainability: Can the system explain why it generated a specific alert or recommendation in clinical terms? Black-box AI is unacceptable in clinical settings
- Bias disclosure: vendor must provide subgroup performance data across gender, age, race/ethnicity, and relevant clinical subgroups, refuse vendors who cannot or will not provide this
- Post-market support: defined process for performance monitoring, adverse event reporting, model updates, and regulatory change communication
- Financial stability and longevity: AI vendor landscape is consolidating rapidly, evaluate vendor stability. What happens to your patient data and clinical workflows if the vendor is acquired or fails?

- Reference sites: speak directly with clinical leaders (not just IT leads) at comparable organisations currently using the system, ask specifically about alert fatigue, workflow integration, and governance support

★ KEY TAKEAWAYS

1. Most AI implementations fail not because the technology does not work, but because implementation is technology-first, without readiness assessment, training, governance, or change management.
2. The Readiness Assessment (six dimensions, scored 1–3) determines whether an organisation is ready to begin Phase 1, needs foundational work, or must defer AI implementation entirely.
3. The four-phase roadmap, Awareness, Training, Pilot, Scale, must be followed in sequence. Each phase has defined entry criteria, key actions, success metrics, and risk mitigations.
4. Use case prioritisation: start with high-impact, lower-complexity AI (sepsis alerts, radiology AI, medication safety); build to moderate complexity; plan for transformative applications.
5. Vendor selection is a patient safety decision, nine non-negotiable criteria including clinical evidence, regulatory status, bias disclosure, explainability, and reference site validation.
6. Bhagyoday's sequencing lesson: deploy low-risk AI first, learn from it, build governance confidence, then scale to clinical AI. The discipline of sequencing produces the trust that enables transformation.

▶ COMING NEXT

Chapter 20 addresses the most human dimension of AI implementation, change management. Technology can be deployed. People must be led. This chapter provides the specific tools, frameworks, and leadership approaches that convert resistance into adoption and adoption into sustained excellence.

Chapter 20

Change Management in Hospitals

Overcoming Resistance, Leading Transformation, and Building the Culture That Makes AI Work

> *"Culture eats strategy for breakfast."*
>
> **Peter Drucker in healthcare AI, the most sophisticated strategy, the most validated algorithm, and the most generous budget are all consumed by culture if culture is not addressed first.**

20.1 Introduction: Technology Is the Easy Part

If healthcare leaders could change one misconception about AI implementation, it would be this: the technology is not the hard part. Selecting a validated AI system, configuring its integration with the EHR, establishing the governance framework, and training staff on how to use the system, these are complex tasks, but they are manageable tasks. They follow a sequence. They have defined endpoints. They can be planned, budgeted, and executed.

The hard part, the part that determines whether an AI implementation succeeds or fails in real clinical practice, is human. It is the physician who says, 'I've been doing this for twenty years and I don't need a computer to tell me what to do.' It is the nurse who, under pressure at 3 AM, stops checking the AI alert because it has cried wolf seventeen times already this week. It is the administrator who approved the AI budget but never championed it publicly. It is the institutional culture that rewards moving fast over moving carefully, that treats failure as weakness rather than learning, and that has never developed the psychological safety that genuine improvement requires.

Change management is the discipline that addresses the human dimension of transformation. It is not soft or peripheral; it is central and determinative. This chapter provides healthcare leaders with the specific frameworks, tools, and leadership approaches that convert resistance to adoption and adoption to sustained cultural transformation.

20.2 Understanding Resistance: The Leader's Essential Competency

Before resistance can be addressed, it must be understood. Healthcare leaders who treat resistance as an irrational obstruction that must be overcome miss the most important signal that resistance carries: information about what is actually needed for successful implementation.

Resistance in healthcare is almost always rational from the perspective of the person resisting. The physician who resists AI is often protecting something real: their professional identity, their clinical judgment, their relationships with patients, their fear of accountability for decisions they feel were made by an algorithm. The nurse who ignores AI alerts has usually done so because the alerts have been unreliable, not because the nurse is negligent. The administrator who deprioritises AI governance has usually done so because they are already managing forty competing priorities, not because they do not care about patient safety.

Understanding the specific root cause of each category of resistance is the precondition for addressing it effectively. Generic 'change management' that treats all resistance as the same phenomenon produces generic results, which is to say, limited results. Precise diagnosis of resistance leads to precisely calibrated responses.

Who Resists	Root Cause of Resistance	What They Fear	Leader's Response
Senior Physicians	Loss of professional authority and identity, 'AI is replacing my expertise'	Being seen as unnecessary, replaceable, or less capable than an algorithm	Involve senior physicians as AI evaluators and governance leaders from the very beginning; never as recipients of decisions made by others. Frame AI as enhancing their capability, never replacing their judgment
Junior Doctors / Residents	Uncertainty about how to use AI in practice, 'What if I disagree with the AI and I'm wrong?'	Making an error by overriding AI and being blamed; or making an error by following AI without thinking	Provide explicit training on how to engage critically with AI; create safe practice environments; establish clear documentation standards for AI disagreement; make critical AI use explicitly valued
Nursing Staff	Alert fatigue and workflow disruption, 'This AI makes more work, not less'	Being blamed for missing an AI alert; or wasting time on false positive alerts that have no clinical consequence	Involve nurses in alert threshold calibration; take alert fatigue seriously and fix it; design AI workflows that reduce documentation burden; celebrate

			nursing-identified AI improvements
Hospital Administrators	ROI uncertainty and competing priorities, 'We spent this money and I cannot show the board what we got'	Being accountable for a large investment that does not deliver; disrupting operations in ways that affect revenue	Provide specific financial projections (readmission reduction, LOS reduction, coding accuracy); set realistic timelines; give administrators visible roles in AI governance
IT Department	Technical complexity and accountability without authority, 'We are responsible for a system we did not choose'	Being blamed for AI failures that arise from clinical configuration decisions made without IT input	Involve IT in vendor selection from the beginning; establish clear accountability boundaries; invest in IT team AI technical training; give IT formal representation in AI governance
Patients and Community	Privacy concerns and loss of human connection, 'I don't want a computer making decisions about my care'	Loss of privacy; being reduced to a data point; receiving care that feels inhuman or opaque	Develop patient AI transparency statement; obtain meaningful informed consent; ensure patients know AI supports but never replaces physician judgment; provide opt-out information

20.3 The Kotter 8-Step Change Model: Applied to Healthcare AI

John Kotter's 8-Step Change Model, developed at Harvard Business School, is the most widely validated framework for leading complex organisational transformation. Each of its eight steps maps directly onto the challenges of healthcare AI adoption, and each step is a place where leadership either builds momentum or loses it.

Step 1	CREATE URGENCY: Build a compelling case for change that connects AI implementation to patient outcomes, competitive position, financial sustainability, and the values of the organisation. Use data, patient harm events that AI could have prevented, efficiency gaps quantified in lost time and revenue, and competitor activity. Leaders who skip this step create implementation programmes that lack the organisational energy to sustain themselves through the inevitable difficulties of change.
Step 2	BUILD A GUIDING COALITION: Assemble a cross-functional team of respected leaders: clinical, administrative, technical, and patient representative, who champion the AI transformation from positions of genuine authority and credibility. A coalition built on formal authority alone will not survive the first serious challenge. A coalition built on respected leaders who are genuinely convinced that AI transformation is right will.
Step 3	FORM A STRATEGIC VISION: Develop a clear, specific vision of what the AI-transformed hospital looks and feels like, not just in technical terms but in patient experience terms. 'We will be a hospital where no patient deteriorates without our clinical team knowing in advance and being able to intervene' is a vision. 'We will implement five AI systems by 2027' is a project plan. Visions inspire. Project plans do not.
Step 4	ENLIST A VOLUNTEER ARMY: Identify and develop AI champions at every level of the organisation, the enthusiastic physician who wants to be involved, the tech-savvy nurse manager, the data analyst who understands quality improvement. These champions are the multiplying force of change. They reach colleagues that

	senior leaders cannot reach. They translate AI from abstract to concrete in the language their peers understand.
Step 5	ENABLE ACTION BY REMOVING BARRIERS: Identify and systematically remove the structural, process, and resource barriers that prevent staff from engaging with AI. Alert fatigue is a barrier, fix it. Insufficient training time is a barrier, create it. Unclear accountability is a barrier, define it. A change management programme that identifies barriers but does not remove them teaches staff that the barriers are actually the point.
Step 6	GENERATE SHORT-TERM WINS: Identify and celebrate specific, visible, credible early wins from AI implementation, before the broader transformation is complete. A 30% reduction in time-to-sepsis-antibiotic in the pilot ward. A 40% reduction in medication documentation time on one unit. These wins serve two purposes: they demonstrate that the vision is achievable, and they provide evidence that counters resistance from sceptics who doubt that AI delivers real value.
Step 7	SUSTAIN ACCELERATION: Use the credibility of early wins to expand the change, more departments, more AI applications, deeper integration. Avoid declaring victory too early. The most dangerous moment in healthcare AI transformation is after the first visible success, when leadership attention moves to the next priority, and the transformation is left to sustain itself without continued leadership investment.
Step 8	INSTITUTE CHANGE: Anchor AI transformation in the culture, through hiring practices that value AI literacy, performance management that includes AI engagement, leadership development that builds change management capability, and explicit institutional narratives that celebrate innovation and continuous improvement. Culture change is complete when the new way of working is how things are done here, not how things were changed here.

20.4 Leadership Role in AI Transformation: The Five Imperatives

Leadership in AI transformation is not about being the most knowledgeable person in the room about AI technology. It is about creating the conditions under which transformation can succeed. The following five leadership imperatives are non-negotiable for any leader driving healthcare AI adoption:

The Five Leadership Imperatives for AI Transformation

- IMPERATIVE 1, VISIBLE COMMITMENT: Leaders must be seen, not just heard, championing AI transformation. This means attending implementation events, reviewing AI performance dashboards personally, asking questions about AI results in management meetings, and publicly acknowledging both successes and problems. Invisible leadership produces invisible change
- IMPERATIVE 2, PSYCHOLOGICAL SAFETY: Leaders must create the environment in which staff feel safe to express concerns about AI, report AI performance issues, and say 'I overrode the AI recommendation because...' without fear of punishment. The leader who responds to AI concerns with defensiveness teaches staff to hide concerns. The leader who responds with genuine curiosity teaches staff to surface them
- IMPERATIVE 3, RESOURCE COMMITMENT: AI transformation requires real investment, in training time, governance infrastructure, data quality improvement, and change management support. Leaders who announce AI transformation without allocating the resources it requires create the cynicism that is the hardest form of resistance to overcome
- IMPERATIVE 4, PATIENCE WITH PROCESS: AI transformation takes longer than technology deployment. Leaders must protect the implementation process from the pressure to rush, from boards that want results now, from vendors that promise faster deployment, from internal critics who want to skip governance steps. The leader who protects the process protects the transformation

- IMPERATIVE 5, ACCOUNTABILITY WITHOUT BLAME: When AI implementation encounters difficulties, and it will, leaders must respond with the same accountability-without-blame approach that effective quality management requires. Investigate root causes. Fix systems. Learn publicly. Blame privately if at all. The leader who publicly blames individuals for AI implementation difficulties will find that the next problem is hidden rather than surfaced

20.5 Culture Transformation: Making AI the Way Things Are Done Here

The goal of change management in healthcare AI is not adoption; it is culture transformation. Adoption means staff use AI tools when they are required to. Culture transformation means staff embrace AI tools because they have experienced that AI tools make them better at what they care about: providing excellent care to their patients.

The difference matters enormously for sustainability. Adopted AI is vulnerable to the next leadership transition, the next budget pressure, and the next technology trend. Culturally embedded AI is resilient, because it has become part of how the organisation understands itself.

Culture transformation in healthcare AI requires three things to happen simultaneously: staff experience AI as genuinely helpful to their clinical work; the institution's formal systems (training requirements, performance management, governance) signal that AI engagement is a professional expectation; and leaders visibly model the behaviours they are asking of staff, using AI tools, reviewing AI performance data, participating in AI governance, and speaking with genuine conviction about why AI transformation matters for their patients.

Signals That Culture Is Transforming	Warning Signs of Adoption Without Culture	Culture Intervention Tools
• Clinical staff spontaneously share AI learnings with colleagues • Staff identify and report AI performance issues through governance channels • AI is discussed in clinical handover as part of normal information sharing • Staff request better AI tools for problems they identify in their work • New staff cite AI capability as a reason for choosing your institution • AI performance is a standing agenda item in departmental quality meetings • Patient satisfaction surveys mention AI-supported care positively	• AI alerts are routinely dismissed without review after first weeks • Staff bypass AI tools whenever possible • AI is only discussed in formal governance meetings, not clinical conversations • Staff cannot explain why AI recommendations differ from their own judgment • New staff are never introduced to AI tools as part of onboarding • AI errors are hidden rather than reported • Leadership champions left the building and AI usage declined	• AI champions programme, peer-to-peer AI support embedded in every department • AI learning huddles, brief weekly team discussions of AI performance and learning • Recognition programme, celebrate staff who use AI to improve patient care • AI improvement suggestions system, structured pathway for staff to suggest AI improvements • Leadership AI rounds, senior leaders visit clinical areas to discuss AI in practice • AI onboarding, every new staff member receives AI orientation in Week 1

		• AI performance storytelling, share specific patient stories where AI made a difference

★ KEY TAKEAWAYS

7. Technology is the easy part, human resistance, cultural inertia, and leadership consistency determine whether AI implementation succeeds or fails in practice.
8. Resistance is always rational from the perspective of the person resisting, diagnose its specific root cause before designing the response. Generic change management produces generic results.
9. The six categories of healthcare AI resistance, physicians, junior doctors, nurses, administrators, IT, and patients, each require specifically calibrated engagement and response strategies.
10. Kotter's 8-Step Change Model provides the leadership framework: urgency, coalition, vision, champions, barrier removal, early wins, sustained momentum, and cultural embedding.
11. Five leadership imperatives are non-negotiable: visible commitment, psychological safety, resource commitment, patience with process, and accountability without blame.
12. The goal is culture transformation, not adoption, AI embedded in how things are done here, not imposed as a requirement. The difference determines sustainability across leadership transitions.
13. Transparency about problems builds more trust than perfection, Bhagyoday's experience demonstrates that openly addressed AI failures strengthen confidence in the governance system.

▶ COMING NEXT

Chapter 21 brings the Bhagyoday case study

Chapter 21

Case Study: Bhagyoday Hospital and Medical College

Vision, Phases, Implementation and Lessons can be applied to Build a World-Class Healthcare in Kadi, Gujarat.

21.1 Introduction: Why Bhagyoday Matters Beyond Gujarat

Bhagyoday Hospital and Medical College in Kadi, Gujarat, is not simply a local healthcare facility.

Kadi is a town with a population of approximately 50,000 in Gujarat's Mehsana district, approximately 50 kilometers north of Ahmedabad. The surrounding region, predominantly agricultural, with significant socioeconomic diversity, represents the patient population that Bhagyoday was built to serve: families who deserve world-class healthcare and have previously had access only to fragmented, resource-constrained services in either Kadi's limited facilities or the overloaded government and private hospitals of Ahmedabad.

The Bhagyoday model is built on a conviction: geography should not determine health outcomes. That a farmer in Kadi who presents with chest pain should receive care of equal quality to an executive in Ahmedabad. That a medical student in Kadi should receive education of equal rigour to a student at a metropolitan medical college. And that artificial intelligence, quality management, and human values, applied together with genuine leadership commitment, can make this equality of excellence a reality, not just an aspiration.

21.2 The proposed Implementation Phases

Phase 1, Foundation

Key Initiatives

- Vision articulation and stakeholder alignment, board, medical leadership, community
- Site assessment and infrastructure planning to make SMART buildings: location, utilities, network architecture
- NABH gap analysis against vision standards, design for world class
- EHR vendor selection, ABDM-compliant, FHIR R4 native, AI integration-ready
- Faculty recruitment, clinical expertise AND teaching philosophy assessed in every appointment
- AI & Ethics Committee formation
- Community engagement, patient advisory group established
- Simulation centre design, curriculum-integrated, not compliance checkbox
- Staff AI literacy curriculum design, role-specific, practical, locally relevant

Phase 2, Digital Infrastructure

Key Initiatives

- EHR go-live, all clinical departments; zero paper clinical records from Day 1
- Medical device integration, all ICU monitors, lab analyzers, radiology (DICOM/PACS) connected to EHR
- ABHA Health ID creation, standard practice at registration for all patients
- Laboratory Information System (LIS) integration, results delivered electronically within 30 minutes
- Radiology PACS deployment, all imaging digital, AI-ready
- Pharmacy management system, barcode dispensing and medication reconciliation
- Staff AI literacy training, Phase 1 (foundational) completed for all 200 staff
- Data quality audit, first formal assessment at 6 months post-opening

Phase 4, Expansion and Accreditation	
Key Initiatives	**Outcomes Achieved**
• Sepsis AI expansion, all inpatient wards; updated bias audit shows equitable performance across patient demographics • Predictive readmission AI, discharge planning integration; high-risk patients identified for follow-up • Full NABH accreditation survey, comprehensive 3-day assessment • NMC medical college accreditation visit, CBME implementation reviewed; AI literacy in curriculum assessed • AI-integrated ward rounds, clinical dashboard showing patient risk scores, pending investigations, and AI alerts • Community health AI, telemedicine deployment for village health outreach; AI triage support • Research programme launch, three faculty-led AI clinical research projects submitted to ICMR • Bhagyoday Model documentation, formal publication of methodology for national dissemination	14. NABH accreditation achieved, first hospital in Mehsana district 15. NMC accreditation confirmed, CBME AI integration noted as exemplary in assessment report 16. Readmission rate: 8.2% at 30 days (vs. 14.7% pre-AI; national average 13.8%) 17. Sepsis mortality: 18% reduction vs. pre-AI baseline (statistically significant) 18. Telemedicine: 340 village consultations in the first 6 months; 78% avoided unnecessary hospital journey 19. Three research papers submitted; one accepted in the National Medical Journal of India

21.4 What Every Leader Must Know

This journey will produce hard-won lessons that are more valuable than any theoretical framework.

Lesson 1	START WITH THE PATIENT, NOT THE TECHNOLOGY. Every technology decision began with a patient question: what would this patient experience be if this technology worked perfectly? What would be lost if this technology failed? This framing kept the focus on patient outcomes rather than technology specifications and produced systems that clinicians actually used because they could see their value to patients.
Lesson 2	DATA QUALITY IS NOT AN IT PROBLEM; IT IS A CLINICAL CULTURE PROBLEM. The 6-month data quality audit revealed that the gaps in data completeness were not caused by EHR limitations; they were caused by clinical workflow habits. Physicians completing notes hours after patient contact. Nurses entering observations from memory rather than at point of care. The solution was clinical leadership, not technology: faculty leads who modelled timely documentation and held their teams accountable.
Lesson 3	THE FIRST PROBLEM IS A GIFT. When the sepsis AI alert threshold miscalibrated and produced 3 weeks of false positives, the temptation was to quietly fix it without acknowledgment. The decision was made instead to announce the problem transparently, explain what was being done, and use it as a teaching moment about how AI governance works. The trust this built was more valuable than any suppressed problem could have been.
Lesson 4	CHAMPIONS ARE THE INFRASTRUCTURE OF CHANGE. The physicians, nurses, and administrators become AI champions.
Lesson 5	ACCREDITATION IS A QUALITY IMPROVEMENT TOOL, NOT A COMPLIANCE EXERCISE. The NABH accreditation process should be approached as a rigorous external review of the institution's quality systems, not as a documentation exercise to satisfy auditors..
Lesson 6	WORLD-CLASS IS ACHIEVABLE. The most important lesson is the simplest: it can be done. A world-class, AI-integrated, NABH-

accredited hospital with a fully digital medical college curriculum can be built. The obstacles, limited resources, geographic constraints, are real but not determinative. What is determinative is vision, values, discipline, and the refusal to accept that excellence is the exclusive privilege of the already-advantaged.

★ KEY TAKEAWAYS

20. AI, Quality & Digital transformation be integrated, patient-centered healthcare is achievable in a semi-urban context with real constraints and real patients.
21. The vision, fully digital, AI-enabled, NABH-accredited, patient-centered, and replicable, must be articulated before any operational decision. Vision governs every subsequent choice.
22. Four implementation phases: Foundation, Digital Infrastructure, First AI Deployments, Expansion and Accreditation, each with specific initiatives and measurable outcomes.
23. Six lessons: start with the patient; data quality is a clinical culture problem; the first problem is a gift; champions are the infrastructure of change; accreditation is a quality tool; world-class is achievable outside metropolitan centers.

▶ COMING NEXT

Part 7, the final part of this book, returns to where it began: the human heart of healthcare. Chapters 22, 23, and 24 address compassion in the digital age, leadership in transformation, and the balanced future where AI and humanity work together in the service of every patient, everywhere.

PART SEVEN

Humanity, Leadership & the Future

Where we return to the beginning, the patient, the healer, and the future they must build together

Chapter 22

Human Values in a Digital World

Compassion in the Age of AI, Protecting What Technology Can Never Replace

> *"The good physician treats the disease. The great physician treats the patient who has the disease."*
>
> **Sir William Osler, whose distinction between treating disease and treating the patient becomes more important, not less, in the era of AI.**

22.1 Introduction: The Paradox of Progress

We have spent this book making the case for artificial intelligence in healthcare, for its diagnostic accuracy, its operational efficiency, its educational power, its regulatory compliance support, and its potential to extend world-class care to patients who currently receive none. That case is sound. The technology is real. The evidence is compelling. The opportunity is historic.

And yet, the more powerful AI becomes in healthcare, the more essential human values become. This is not a paradox. It is a logical consequence of what AI is and what it is not. AI is extraordinary at pattern recognition, at data synthesis, and at consistent application of evidence-based protocols. It is incapable of compassion, of moral judgment, of genuine relationship, of the kind of presence that transforms a clinical encounter from a transaction into a healing experience.

As AI assumes more of the technical cognitive labour of medicine, what remains irreducibly human, what cannot be automated, delegated to an algorithm, or replicated by a machine, becomes more valuable, not less. The physician who brings genuine compassion to the consultation room, who sees the person behind the diagnosis, who communicates with warmth and honesty, who advocates for their patient's dignity, that physician is not replaceable by AI. They are, in the AI era, more indispensable than ever.

This chapter is about protecting and cultivating those irreducibly human dimensions of healthcare, not as an idealistic counterweight to technology, but as the primary professional obligation of every person who works in healthcare. Technology serves humanity. Never the reverse.

22.2 What Compassion Is, and What It Is Not

Compassion is the most misunderstood word in medical education. It is frequently conflated with kindness, with empathy, with niceness, with patient satisfaction scores. These are related but distinct. Compassion, from the Latin compassio, to suffer together, is something more specific and more demanding: it is the recognition of another person's suffering and the genuine motivation to act to relieve it.

Compassion is not a feeling that some people have and others do not. It is not a personality trait that either belongs to you or does not. It is a practice, a set of deliberate attentional and behavioural habits that can be developed, strengthened, and sustained. It is also, as the evidence increasingly demonstrates, a clinical competency: physicians who practice compassion have patients with better adherence, better outcomes, and greater trust. Compassion is not peripheral to clinical effectiveness. It is central to it.

In the AI era, compassion faces a specific threat: the displacement of attention. When a physician is simultaneously managing EHR alerts, AI recommendations, electronic orders, and digital documentation, while trying to be present with a patient who is frightened and in pain, attention becomes the scarcest clinical resource. Protecting the attentional space that compassion requires, designing AI systems that reduce administrative burden precisely so that human attention can go where it cannot be replaced, is one of the most important leadership responsibilities in the digital hospital.

What Compassion Requires	What AI Can Support	What AI Cannot Replace
• Full presence, physically and mentally with the patient, not with the screen • Genuine listening, hearing not just what is said but what is meant • Recognition, seeing the person, not just the diagnosis • Response, acting on what you have understood, not just acknowledging it • Continuity, sustained over time, not performed in single encounters • Reciprocity, allowing the patient's experience to genuinely affect you • Recovery, sustaining compassion under the	• Reducing documentation burden, freeing physician attention for the patient • Flagging patients at risk of deterioration, enabling proactive compassionate intervention • Personalising patient communication materials, in accessible language and preferred format • Scheduling sufficient consultation time, AI scheduling tools that protect relational time • Monitoring staff burnout indicators, enabling proactive wellbeing support • Analysing patient feedback,	• The moment of genuine human recognition, 'I see you, and I care' • The silence after difficult news that says more than words • The touch that communicates what language cannot • The judgment to know when to follow protocol and when to break it for this patient • The moral courage to advocate when advocacy is needed • The relationship that is maintained across years of care • The meaning that makes healing more than the treatment of disease

pressure of clinical work	identifying where compassion is consistently experienced or absent • Supporting family communication, automated updates that maintain connection	

22.3 The Doctor-Patient Relationship in the AI Era

The doctor-patient relationship is the oldest and most powerful therapeutic tool in medicine. Long before antibiotics, before surgery, before imaging, the healer's presence, attention, and genuine care produced measurable therapeutic effects. The placebo effect is not a trick of the mind. It is the clinical expression of human relationship. Hope, trust, and the feeling of being cared for are biologically active. They activate the immune system, modulate the stress response, and improve the physiological conditions in which healing occurs.

AI does not threaten this relationship. But the misuse of AI does. The physician who is so focused on the AI dashboard that they forget to look at the patient. The consultation that is mediated entirely through screens and algorithms with no genuine human contact. The care plan generated by AI and delivered without explanation or dialogue. The diagnosis communicated via automated message rather than a human conversation. These are failures of humanity that technology makes possible but does not require.

Protecting the doctor-patient relationship in the AI era is an active leadership responsibility, not a passive wish. It requires designing AI workflows that serve the relationship rather than disrupting it. It requires training clinicians in the specific skills of maintaining genuine presence in technology-mediated environments. And it requires a cultural commitment, expressed in how performance is measured, how staff are recognised, and what is celebrated, that places human relationship at the center of clinical excellence.

Protecting the Doctor-Patient Relationship, Practical Principles for the Digital Hospital

- Screen-free opening: every consultation begins with 30-60 seconds of full human attention before any screen is opened, establishing the relationship before accessing information
- Eye contact priority: AI dashboards and EHR screens positioned so clinicians can maintain eye contact with patients without turning away, physical design matters
- Narrated documentation: when documentation must occur during the consultation, narrate it, 'I am recording what you have just told me', maintaining transparency and connection
- AI transparency: inform patients when AI is supporting clinical decisions, 'Our system has highlighted something I want to discuss with you', maintains trust and informed consent
- Protected consultation time: AI scheduling systems must protect sufficient time for genuine clinical dialogue, productivity metrics must never be the sole driver of appointment duration
- Family engagement: AI-assisted family communication tools supplement, never replace, direct physician communication about significant diagnoses, deterioration, or end-of-life decisions
- The last question: every consultation ends with 'Is there anything else you wanted to tell me, or anything you are still worried about?', the question that the AI cannot ask and that the physician must never omit

22.4 Preventing Burnout: Sustaining the Human Who Heals

Compassion cannot be sustained by a burned-out clinician. And burnout in healthcare is at epidemic levels. More than 50% of US physicians report symptoms of burnout. Indian physicians in government health systems carry patient loads that are physiologically incompatible with sustained compassionate practice. The irony is sharp: healthcare systems that exhaust their healers in the name of productivity destroy the very human quality that makes healthcare genuinely healing.

AI, properly implemented, can address several root causes of clinician burnout: by reducing administrative documentation burden, by improving the efficiency of clinical workflows, by providing decision support that reduces the cognitive load of complex clinical decisions, and by enabling better scheduling that protects time for recovery. These are real and important contributions. But they are not sufficient.

Sustaining the human who heals also requires institutional cultures that take clinician wellbeing seriously, not as a wellness programme add-on, but as a strategic imperative. That means protected time for reflection and recovery. Peer support systems that allow clinicians to process the emotional weight of their work. Leadership that models healthy professional boundaries. Recognition systems that value the quality of human care, not just the volume of clinical throughput. And the intellectual honesty to acknowledge that no AI system can eliminate the inherent emotional demands of a profession that involves sitting with human suffering every day.

22.5 Human Values as the Anchor of AI Governance

Throughout this book, we have discussed AI governance in technical and regulatory terms: ethics committees, bias auditing, performance monitoring, explainability requirements, and regulatory compliance. All of these are essential. But the deepest anchor of AI governance in healthcare is not regulatory; it is values.

The values of healthcare, the conviction that every patient deserves dignity, the commitment to truth-telling, the obligation to 'first, do no harm', the dedication to equity, the respect for patient autonomy, these are the standards against which every AI system must ultimately be evaluated. Not: 'Does it pass regulatory review?' But: 'Does it treat every patient with the dignity they deserve? Does it tell the clinical team the truth? Does it do no harm to patients of any demographic group, in any clinical context? Does it support equitable care or amplify existing inequities? Does it respect the patient's right to understand and participate in their own care?'

These questions cannot be answered by algorithms. They require human judgment, moral commitment, and the willingness to make difficult decisions, to suspend an AI system that is working well for most patients but failing for some. To invest in bias correction even when the biased system is performing adequately by aggregate metrics. To prioritise the most vulnerable patient over the most efficient process.

Human values are not the soft counterpart to AI's hard capabilities. They are the governance framework within which AI must operate, the non-negotiable conditions on which the promise of AI in healthcare depends.

⋆ KEY TAKEAWAYS

1. The more powerful AI becomes, the more essential human values become: compassion, presence, moral judgment, and genuine relationships are irreplaceable precisely because AI cannot provide them.
2. Compassion is not a personality trait; it is a clinical practice, a learnable competency, and a therapeutic tool whose biological effects on patient outcomes are well-documented.
3. AI can support compassion by reducing administrative burden and freeing clinician attention, but the attentional space that compassion requires must be actively protected in system design.
4. The doctor-patient relationship is the oldest and most powerful therapeutic tool in medicine, protecting it in the AI era requires deliberate design, training, and cultural commitment.

5. Clinician burnout is the greatest threat to sustained compassion in healthcare, AI must address root causes, but institutional culture, leadership modelling, and protected recovery time are equally essential.
6. Human values, dignity, truth, non-maleficence, equity, autonomy, are the deepest anchor of AI governance. Every AI decision must be evaluated against these values, not just against regulatory compliance.

▶ COMING NEXT

Chapter 23 addresses the leadership that brings all of this together, the specific qualities, decisions, and development of the leaders who will determine whether AI transformation in healthcare serves or fails the patients it is meant to help.

Chapter 23

Leadership in Healthcare Transformation

The Qualities, Decisions, and Development of Leaders Who Will Determine the Future of Healthcare

> *"A leader is one who knows the way, goes the way, and shows the way."*
>
> **John C. Maxwell in healthcare AI transformation, all three are required simultaneously: knowing the destination, doing the work personally, and making the path visible to everyone who must walk it.**

23.1 Introduction: Leadership Is the Variable That Determines Everything

In thirty years of consulting with organisations across industries and continents, one truth has emerged with absolute consistency: the quality of leadership is the single most powerful determinant of organisational outcomes. Not the technology. Not the strategy. Not the market. Not the resources. The people who lead.

In healthcare AI transformation, this truth is multiplied. The leader who understands AI governance and has the courage to enforce it prevents patient harm. The leader who builds psychological safety creates a reporting culture that surfaces problems before they become crises. The leader who models intellectual humility demonstrates that admitting uncertainty is a clinical strength rather than a professional weakness. The leader who champions equity ensures that AI systems serve all patients, not just the majority.

This chapter examines what leadership in healthcare AI transformation specifically requires, the qualities that must be developed, the decisions that must be made well, and the approach to building high-performance teams that can sustain transformation over the long timelines it requires.

23.2 The Healthcare Transformation Leader: Essential Qualities

Leadership in healthcare AI transformation requires a specific combination of qualities that is rare in any single individual, and that therefore must be developed deliberately, across careers, through experience, mentorship, and structured leadership development.

Vision Clarity	The transformation leader sees, with genuine precision, not vague aspiration, what the transformed organisation will look like, feel like, and deliver for patients. They can articulate this vision in terms that resonate with a frontline nurse, a board member, a patient's family, and a data scientist simultaneously. This is not a communication skill. It is a clarity of purpose that comes from having genuinely worked through the implications of the transformation, its costs, its benefits, its timeline, its risks, and its irreversible commitments.
Intellectual Humility	The greatest danger in healthcare AI leadership is the confident incompetence of leaders who believe they understand AI better than they do, who make confident procurement, deployment, and governance decisions based on vendor presentations rather than genuine understanding. Intellectual humility, the ability to say 'I need to understand this more deeply before I decide', is a leadership strength that protects patients from the consequences of overconfident decision-making.
Moral Courage	Healthcare AI transformation will produce moments that require leaders to do difficult things: suspend a popular AI system because its bias audit failed; tell a vendor that their system is underperforming and must be recalibrated; override a financially attractive AI contract because the governance terms are inadequate; publish an AI performance failure publicly when transparency is the right response. Moral courage, doing the right thing when it is

	costly, is the leadership quality that distinguishes transformation from performance.
Systemic Thinking	Healthcare is a system of systems: clinical, educational, regulatory, technological, financial, cultural, and AI transformation interacts with all of them simultaneously. The leader who addresses AI implementation as a technology project misses the systemic reverberations: the effect on clinical workflow, the impact on staff wellbeing, the regulatory implications, the patient experience consequences, the cultural signals. Systemic thinking, the ability to see second and third-order effects of decisions, is indispensable in healthcare transformation leadership.
People Development	No single leader can sustain a healthcare AI transformation alone. The transformation requires developing leaders at every level, clinical champions, department heads, quality managers, IT leaders, patient advocates, who can drive the change in their specific domains. The transformation leader who does not develop others is building a dependency that will collapse when they leave. The transformational leader who develops others is building an institution.

23.3 High-Performance Teams in the AI-Integrated Hospital

The AI-integrated hospital requires teams that are different from the hierarchical clinical teams of the 20th century, teams that are genuinely interprofessional rather than traditionally hierarchical, that use data to drive decisions rather than authority and intuition, that maintain psychological safety to surface problems, and that develop AI literacy across all roles rather than concentrating it in specialist functions.

Building these teams is a leadership responsibility that requires explicit attention. High-performance teams in the AI era share five defining characteristics that distinguish them from merely competent groups of capable individuals:

- Shared purpose that is larger than role: every team member, from the physician to the data analyst to the ward administrator, understands and is genuinely committed to the patient outcome the team exists to achieve. AI tools are used because team members believe they improve that outcome, not because they are required to.

- Psychological safety without complacency: team members feel safe raising concerns about AI performance, questioning clinical decisions, and reporting near-misses, but also hold each other to high standards of performance and continuous improvement. Psychological safety is not the absence of accountability. It is the presence of trust.

- Data literacy at every level: every team member can read and interpret the data that governs their work, whether that is the AI performance dashboard for a nurse manager, the bias audit results for a department head, or the outcome data for a frontline clinician. Data-literate teams make better decisions and hold AI systems to higher standards.

- Disciplined learning: every team has a structured approach to learning from both successes and failures, through regular debriefs, quality improvement projects, AI performance reviews, and explicit celebration of learning. High-performance teams do not just perform. They get better.

- Adaptive leadership: authority in the high-performance team shifts to the most knowledgeable person for the problem at hand, not the most senior person. The junior doctor who has the most current evidence leads the evidence discussion. The nurse who has observed the patient most closely leads the deterioration discussion. The AI champion leads the AI calibration discussion. Hierarchy serves coordination, not decision quality.

23.4 Leadership Decision-Making in Transformational Contexts

Transformational leadership requires decision-making under conditions of genuine uncertainty, about technology performance, about organisational readiness, about staff capacity, about patient outcomes, and about the regulatory landscape. Leaders who wait for certainty before deciding are not being cautious. They are being ineffective. The decisions that matter most in healthcare AI transformation are the ones that must be made before the evidence is complete.

The framework for good decision-making under uncertainty in healthcare AI transformation has five components: clear values that anchor decisions when data is ambiguous; structured information gathering that goes beyond vendor claims to clinical evidence, reference sites, and independent expert advice; genuine consultation with the people who will be affected by the decision; explicit acknowledgment of uncertainty in communication with stakeholders; and commitment to monitoring and adjustment once the decision is made. This is not indecisiveness. It is intellectual honesty combined with disciplined action.

The Leadership Decision Framework for Healthcare AI, Five Questions
• Values question: Is this decision consistent with our commitment to patient safety, equity, dignity, and transparency? If any of these values is compromised by this decision, the decision requires fundamental reconsideration, not just better communication • Evidence question: What does the best available evidence say about this AI system's performance in populations like ours? Have we verified vendor claims independently? Have we spoken with clinical leaders at reference sites who have no commercial interest in our decision? • Stakeholder question: Who will be affected by this decision, patients, clinicians, staff, community, and have we genuinely

consulted them? Not informed them after the decision was made, but engaged them in the process of making it?

- Risk question: What are the realistic worst-case scenarios, for patients, for staff, for the institution, if this decision is wrong? Are we prepared to manage those risks? Do we have monitoring systems that will detect problems early enough to respond?
- Learning question: How will we know whether this decision was right? What metrics will we track? How frequently will we review? And, most importantly, what will we do if the evidence shows we were wrong?

23.5 The Leader as Servant: Healthcare Leadership From the Inside Out

The most enduring and most effective model of leadership in healthcare, and in healthcare AI transformation, is servant leadership: the understanding that the leader's role is to create the conditions under which the people they lead can do their best work for the patients they serve.

Servant leadership in the AI era is not a weakness. It is the most sophisticated form of institutional effectiveness. The servant leader who invests in staff training before deploying AI tools is creating the conditions for adoption. The servant leader who removes the bureaucratic barriers that prevent clinical staff from engaging with AI governance is creating the conditions for participation. The servant leader who takes the first step in admitting 'I was wrong about this and here is what I am doing about it' is creating the conditions for the psychological safety that improvement requires.

The servant leader is also, ultimately, the one who builds institutions that outlast their own leadership, because they have developed the next generation of leaders, embedded the values in the culture, and created systems that continue to improve regardless of who is at the top. This is the legacy that healthcare transformation requires: not a dependency on a visionary individual, but institutions that embody the vision in every role, every system, and every patient encounter.

From the village of Thol to the vision of Bhagyoday, the journey of this book has always been about service. Service to patients who deserve better. Service to students who deserve more. Service to communities that deserve world-class healthcare. And the role of every leader described in these pages is, finally, the same: to serve those who cannot fully serve themselves, with the best knowledge, the best technology, and the most genuine human compassion that can be brought to bear.

★ KEY TAKEAWAYS

7. Leadership quality is the single most powerful determinant of organisational outcomes, in healthcare AI transformation, the leader's decisions determine whether AI serves or fails patients.
8. Five essential qualities: Vision Clarity, Intellectual Humility, Moral Courage, Systemic Thinking, and People Development, all developable, all requiring deliberate cultivation.
9. High-performance teams in the AI era share five characteristics: shared purpose, psychological safety with accountability, data literacy, disciplined learning, and adaptive leadership.
10. Good decision-making under uncertainty requires five anchors: values clarity, independent evidence, genuine stakeholder consultation, honest acknowledgment of uncertainty, and committed monitoring.
11. Servant leadership, creating conditions for others to do their best work, is the most sophisticated and most durable form of leadership in healthcare AI transformation.
12. The legacy of transformational leadership is not dependency on the visionary individual; it is institutions that embody the vision in every role, every system, and every patient encounter.

▶ COMING NEXT

Chapter 24, the final chapter of this book, looks to the future: the balanced model where AI and humanity work together, the global vision for healthcare transformation, and the invitation to every reader to take their part in building the healthcare system the world needs.

Chapter 24

The Future: AI + Humanity Together

The Balanced Model, the Global Vision, and the Invitation to Build

> *"The best time to plant a tree was twenty years ago. The second best time is now."*
>
> **Ancient proverb the healthcare transformation this book describes could have begun twenty years ago. It begins today, wherever you are, with the decisions you make next.**

24.1 Where We Have Come From: A Summary of the Journey

From beginning, this book has travelled through the purpose and promise of healthcare (Part 1), through the technology that is transforming it (Part 2), through the quality systems that make excellence sustainable (Part 3), through the regulatory and ethical frameworks that make it safe (Part 4), through the medical education that produces the physicians who will deliver it (Part 5), through the implementation practices that make the vision real (Part 6), and now to the future it is all building toward.

That future is not abstract. It is specific. It is a world in which AI helps a nurse in Kadi detect sepsis in a patient who would otherwise deteriorate and die before a physician arrives. In which a medical student in Gujarat learns anatomy with the same richness of simulation technology as a student at Harvard. In which a patient in rural Maharashtra receives a teleconsultation from a specialist in Mumbai, supported by AI triage and AI-enhanced clinical assessment. In which the gap between world-class care and underserved care narrows, not because of charity, but because of technology, quality management, and genuine leadership commitment to equity.

That future is being built, imperfectly, with setbacks, with hard-won lessons, and with the kind of persistent commitment to a long-term vision that is the hallmark of genuine leadership. It is being built at institutions across India, the United States, and the world. And it is waiting to be built wherever you lead.

24.2 The Balanced Model: Technology Serving Humanity

The central argument of this book can be stated simply: AI and humanity are not competitors in healthcare. They are partners. Each brings capabilities the other lacks. Together they create something that neither can achieve alone.

What AI Brings	What Humanity Brings
Pattern recognition at scale, across millions of cases simultaneously	Wisdom, knowing when the pattern does not apply to this patient
Consistency, the same quality of analysis at 3 AM as at 9 AM	Adaptability, responding to the novel, the unexpected, the unprecedented
Speed, processing complex data in milliseconds	Judgment, weighing incommensurable values in irreducible complexity
Memory; never forgetting a guideline, a drug interaction, a prior result	Intuition, the clinical sense that something is wrong before the data confirms it
Objectivity, applying evidence without the distortions of mood or fatigue	Compassion, the motivation to act in the patient's interest that no algorithm can simulate
Scale, serving millions simultaneously without degradation of performance	Relationship, the unique bond between this healer and this patient
Continuous learning, improving with every case across every deployment	Moral agency, accepting responsibility for decisions and their consequences

The balanced model is not a compromise between AI capability and human values. It is the synthesis in which AI amplifies human capability precisely where human beings are limited, and human beings govern, guide, and give meaning to AI precisely where algorithms are incapable. The physician who uses AI to detect what they might miss, and uses their human judgment and compassion to do what AI cannot, is the physician of the future. The hospital that uses AI to improve the efficiency and consistency of care, and uses its human culture and values to ensure that every patient is treated with dignity, is the hospital of the future.

24.3 The Global Vision: What the World Needs Healthcare to Become

The global vision of this book is simple and ambitious: a world in which every person, regardless of geography, income, gender, caste, language, or any other dimension of identity, has access to safe, effective, compassionate, and continuously improving healthcare.

AI makes this vision achievable in ways that were not possible a decade ago. It can extend specialist expertise to rural areas through telemedicine and AI-assisted triage. It can reduce the cost of high-quality care through operational efficiency without reducing the quality of the care itself. It can personalise treatment to the individual patient's biology, preferences, and circumstances in ways that population-level protocols cannot. It can accelerate drug discovery, reduce diagnostic delay, and enable preventive interventions that catch disease before it becomes acute.

But AI alone cannot deliver this vision. It requires leaders with the courage to invest in AI governance rather than just AI technology. It requires educators with the commitment to build the physicians of the future rather than simply training the physicians of the past. It requires policymakers with the wisdom to regulate AI in ways that protect patients without stifling the innovation that patients need. It requires communities with the trust to engage with AI-integrated healthcare as partners rather than subjects. And it requires every healthcare professional, every physician, nurse, administrator, student, and teacher, to hold both the technology and the humanity simultaneously, without letting the excitement of the former diminish the necessity of the latter.

24.4 The Invitation: What You Must Do Now

This book has given you a framework, seven parts, twenty-four chapters, hundreds of specific tools, frameworks, and examples, for understanding, planning, and implementing AI transformation in healthcare. But a framework becomes a legacy only when someone decides to act on it.

The invitation of this final chapter is specific and personal. Wherever you lead, whatever institution, whatever country, whatever role, there are decisions you can make today that move healthcare toward the world described in this book. They do not all require large budgets or executive authority. Many of the most important ones require only commitment.

The Call to Action, What Every Leader Can Do Today

- If you lead a hospital: Begin the AI Readiness Assessment in Chapter 19. Identify one high-impact, lower-complexity AI application to pilot within 12 months. Establish an AI Ethics Committee before deploying the first AI system. Start a soft skills programme for your clinical staff this year
- If you lead a medical college: Review your curriculum against the world-class criteria in Chapter 17A. Identify one evidence-based soft skill teaching method to introduce this academic year. Begin AI literacy training for faculty before attempting AI integration in the student curriculum
- If you are a physician or nurse: Commit to critically evaluating every AI recommendation you receive, not accepting or rejecting it reflexively, but asking why it was generated and whether it is right for this patient. Report one AI performance concern through your institution's governance channel this year
- If you are a medical student: Begin building your personal learning system today, not for examinations, but for the 40-year career of continuous learning that starts the day you graduate. Ask your faculty how they are integrating AI into their clinical practice, and if they are not, ask why not

- If you are a healthcare policymaker: Accelerate the regulatory frameworks that allow safe AI innovation in healthcare, ABDM implementation, CDSCO AI device guidance, FDA AI action plan. Invest in the quality infrastructure that AI requires: EHR adoption, data standards, and workforce AI literacy
- If you are a patient or community member: Ask your healthcare providers how AI is being used in your care. Request the transparency that the Patient AI Charter promises. Participate in patient advisory processes that shape how AI is governed in the institutions that serve your community
- If you are an educator at any level: Teach the human values that no AI can replace: compassion, integrity, service, and the conviction that every human being deserves dignity, with the same rigour that you teach the technical competencies that AI will augment

24.5 A Final Word

That belief, that transformation is always possible with the right knowledge, discipline, and values, has guided thirty years of work with organisations across the world. And it now guides this book, and the hope that the principles described in these pages will spread through the leaders who read them, the institutions that apply them, and the patients whose lives they ultimately improve.

The technology is extraordinary. The regulatory frameworks are increasingly sound. The quality management tools are proven. The educational models are clear. What remains, always, is the human decision to act. To lead. To invest. To build. To care.

Healthcare stands at a moment of transformation unlike any in its history. Artificial intelligence will change how we diagnose, treat, educate, and manage care at a scale that is genuinely historic. But it is human leadership and human values that will determine whether that transformation serves all of humanity or only some of it. Whether it produces physicians who are complete human beings or merely efficient diagnosticians. Whether it builds hospitals that patients trust or systems that patients endure.

The choice is ours. Every day. In every decision. For every patient.

Let us choose well.

> **Technology empowers. Quality ensures excellence. Humanity remains at the center.**
>
> **Jay P. Patel**

Appendix A

AI Implementation Checklist

This checklist supports hospital leaders through the four phases of AI implementation. Use it as a working document, assign owners to each item, track completion, and review in governance meetings. A checked box represents completed action with documented evidence, not simply intention.

PHASE 1, AWARENESS CHECKLIST
Leadership and Governance
[ ] Senior leadership AI education workshop completed (CEO, CMO, CNO, CFO, Board)
[ ] AI champion role defined and champion identified in each clinical department
[ ] AI Ethics Committee formed, all required roles represented, including patient representative
[ ] AI Ethics Committee charter drafted, reviewed, and formally approved
[ ] AI governance policy drafted for committee review
[ ] AI strategy document: 3 priority use cases identified and formally approved by leadership
Staff Education
[ ] AI awareness training designed, role-specific modules for clinical, nursing, administrative, IT staff
[ ] AI awareness training delivered, completion rate >95% documented
[ ] AI literacy assessment completed, baseline competency measured before and after training
[ ] Patient AI transparency statement drafted and approved by patient advisory group
Baseline Assessment

[ ] Current state assessment completed: data quality, workflow mapping, vendor landscape
[ ] EHR readiness for AI assessed, FHIR API availability, data completeness, structured data %
[ ] Medical device integration status assessed by department, all device digital output documented
[ ] KPI baseline documented for all priority AI use case areas
[ ] Budget allocated for Phase 2 activities

PHASE 2, TRAINING CHECKLIST
Vendor Selection
[ ] Formal RFP issued for priority AI application, scoring criteria defined before RFP release
[ ] Clinical evidence reviewed: peer-reviewed validation studies on comparable populations
[ ] FDA clearance / CDSCO registration / CE Marking status independently verified
[ ] Bias disclosure obtained: subgroup performance data across gender, age, race/ethnicity
[ ] BAA / GDPR SCCs / DPDPA compliance agreements executed before any patient data shared
[ ] HL7 FHIR R4 API support technically verified by the IT team in the test environment
[ ] Explainability requirement verified: system can explain specific recommendations in clinical terms
[ ] Reference site calls completed: spoke directly with clinical leaders (not just IT) at comparable organisations
[ ] Financial stability assessment of vendor completed
[ ] Contract executed, including performance guarantees, SLAs, and post-market support terms
Pre-Deployment Validation and Training

[ ] Local validation study protocol designed and ethics-approved
[ ] Local validation study completed: sensitivity, specificity, PPV, NPV on local population documented
[ ] Local validation results reviewed by AI Ethics Committee, formal deployment approval issued
[ ] System-specific training designed, role-specific, hands-on, realistic scenarios
[ ] System-specific training delivered: >95% completion by all pilot site staff
[ ] Clinical champion intensive training completed
[ ] Downtime procedures written, reviewed, and tested
[ ] EHR integration tested in staging environment for a minimum of 4 weeks
[ ] Alert threshold configuration reviewed by the clinical team before go-live
[ ] Go-live communication sent to all pilot site staff and relevant patients

PHASE 3, PILOT CHECKLIST
Go-Live and Early Monitoring
[ ] Pilot site go-live completed with champion and IT support present on Day 1
[ ] Daily performance dashboard review: first 4 weeks: sensitivity, specificity, alert response rate
[ ] Weekly learning huddles: pilot team meets weekly, issues logged and resolved
[ ] Alert calibration review at 2 weeks, 4 weeks, 8 weeks, thresholds adjusted based on clinical feedback
[ ] Incident tracking: all AI-related concerns documented in the AI incident register
Outcome Measurement and Governance
[ ] Pilot KPIs tracked daily, compared to pre-implementation baseline

[ ] First formal bias audit completed: performance across demographic subgroups documented
[ ] No AI-related adverse events, or if any, root cause analysis completed and documented
[ ] Clinician satisfaction survey administered: target >70% satisfaction
[ ] AI Ethics Committee pilot review: performance data presented, continuation approved
[ ] Expansion plan drafted: criteria for moving to Phase 4 defined and agreed

PHASE 4, SCALE CHECKLIST
Phased Expansion
[ ] Expansion rollout schedule: one department per month: champion and support defined for each
[ ] Peer learning: pilot site champions actively mentoring expansion site champions
[ ] Performance dashboard: all sites reporting to unified quality dashboard
[ ] Quarterly AI governance review: all live systems reviewed by the Ethics Committee
[ ] Annual bias audit: all demographic groups, all live AI systems
[ ] Model drift monitoring protocol implemented, automated performance alerts configured
Sustainability and Public Accountability
[ ] Staff refresher training: annual re-certification programme designed and scheduled
[ ] Annual AI governance report: drafted, reviewed by Ethics Committee, published publicly
[ ] AI system registry maintained: all deployed systems, validation status, performance data documented
[ ] Next use case evaluation: Phase 1–3 process initiated for next priority AI application

[ ] Leadership succession plan: AI governance knowledge documented and transferable

Appendix B

Hospital Readiness Assessment for AI and Digital Transformation

This assessment is designed to be completed by a cross-functional leadership team, not by any single individual. Each dimension should be scored through evidence-based discussion, not optimistic self-assessment. Honest low scores are more valuable than inflated high scores. The assessment should be repeated annually or following significant changes to the organisation's digital infrastructure.

Assessment Area and Questions	Score 1: Not Ready	Score 2: Developing	Score 3: Ready
DIGITAL INFRASTRUCTURE I Is our EHR comprehensive, clean, and AI-ready? I Are all clinical devices digitally integrated? I Do we have FHIR APIs available? I Is our network reliable across all departments?	Paper-based or fragmented digital systems; minimal device integration; no FHIR capability; unreliable network	EHR implemented but data quality issues; some device integration; FHIR in development; network mostly reliable	Comprehensive EHR with clean data; all key devices integrated; FHIR R4 APIs available; reliable network hospital-wide
LEADERSHIP COMMITMENT I Does senior leadership explicitly champion AI? I Is there board-level AI governance? I Is AI in the strategic plan with an allocated budget? I Is there a designated AI strategy leader?	AI not on leadership agenda; no governance, not in strategic plan; no budget; no AI leader designated	Leadership supportive; governance in formation; AI in strategy, but not resourced; AI champion identified but not empowered	CEO/CMO actively championing AI; board AI governance committee active; AI in strategic plan with allocated multi-year budget; CDO or equivalent role filled

STAFF READINESS I Have staff completed AI literacy training? I Are AI champions identified and trained? I Is there a plan for ongoing AI education? I Do clinical staff understand AI governance expectations?	No AI training completed; no champions; no plan; staff unaware of governance expectations	Some training completed; champions identified but not fully trained; plan in draft; governance expectations communicated	Role-specific AI training completed >95%; champions trained and active in all departments; ongoing education plan implemented; governance expectations understood and practiced
QUALITY AND SAFETY SYSTEMS I Do we have a functioning quality management system? I Is there a patient safety reporting culture? I Are performance KPIs measured and reviewed regularly? I Do we have Lean Six Sigma capability?	No formal quality system; blame culture; minimal measurement; no improvement methodology	Basic quality system; some safety reporting; measurement ad hoc; improvement methodology awareness	Robust QMS; blame-free safety reporting culture; comprehensive KPI measurement and review; active Lean Six Sigma programme
GOVERNANCE AND ETHICS I Have we established an AI Ethics Committee? I Do we have a written AI governance policy? I Have we defined a bias auditing protocol? I Is there a patient AI transparency statement?	No governance structure; no policy; no bias protocol; no patient transparency	Governance committee forming; policy in draft; bias protocol conceptual; patient transparency in development	AI Ethics Committee active with all required roles; an approved governance policy; a bias auditing protocol defined and implemented; patient AI transparency statement published
FINANCIAL SUSTAINABILITY I Is AI investment	No multi-year budget; no ROI model; no	One-year budget; basic ROI model; some	Multi-year AI budget approved; validated ROI

budgeted across multiple years? I Have we built a realistic ROI model? I Do we have contingency for implementation challenges? I Is the financial model independent of single AI vendor?	contingency; vendor dependency risk not addressed	contingency; vendor diversity being considered	model with realistic assumptions; contingency reserve established; multi-vendor strategy reduces dependency risk

Scoring Interpretation and Next Steps

- Score 16–18 (Ready): Begin AI implementation following the Phase 1 roadmap in Chapter 19. Your foundation is strong, focus on use case selection and vendor evaluation
- Score 11–15 (Developing): Complete the Not Ready items in your lowest-scoring dimensions before beginning Phase 1. Expect 6–12 months of foundational investment. Identify which dimensions most urgently need attention and assign ownership
- Score 6–10 (Not Ready): Significant foundational work required before any AI deployment. Begin with digital infrastructure and leadership alignment. Attempting AI implementation at this readiness level is the most common cause of failed healthcare AI programmes
- All assessments must be repeated annually, readiness is dynamic, not a one-time achievement. Share results transparently with the AI Ethics Committee and board

Appendix C

AI Risk Register Template

This risk register template should be maintained by the AI Ethics Committee and reviewed quarterly. It covers both deployment-phase risks and ongoing operational risks for all live AI systems. Likelihood and Impact are scored 1–5 (1=rare/negligible, 5=certain/catastrophic). Risk Score = Likelihood × Impact. Scores ≥15 = HIGH (immediate action required); 8–14 = MEDIUM (action within 30 days); <8 = LOW (monitor).

Risk	Description	Likelihood (1-5)	Impact (1-5)	Score	Mitigation Strategy
Data Quality Failure	AI model receives incomplete, inaccurate, or delayed data, producing unreliable recommendations that clinicians act upon	**3**	**5**	**15**	Automated data quality monitoring with daily dashboard review; device integration testing protocol; manual data entry audit programme; defined thresholds for AI system suspension when data quality falls below the minimum standard
Alert Fatigue	High false positive rate causes clinical staff to routinely dismiss AI alerts, including genuine alerts, leading to missed clinical events	**4**	**4**	**16**	Alert threshold calibration at 2, 4, and 8 weeks post-deployment; alert fatigue rate tracked as primary KPI; defined maximum false positive threshold; clinical champion authority to

					request recalibration without escalation
Algorithmic Bias	AI system performs significantly worse for specific patient demographic groups, producing disparate outcomes and perpetuating health inequities	**3**	**5**	**15**	Mandatory pre-deployment bias audit across all demographic subgroups; quarterly re-auditing post-deployment; defined disparity threshold triggering automatic suspension; corrective action protocol with vendor
Model Drift	AI model performance degrades over time as patient population or clinical practice changes, without detection until an adverse outcome occurs	**3**	**4**	**12**	Monthly performance metric review against baseline; automated drift detection alerts configured in AI system; defined performance floor triggering governance review; annual model revalidation requirement
Cybersecurity Breach	Unauthorized access to patient data through AI system interface or training data, compromising patient privacy and institutional integrity	**2**	**5**	**10**	All AI systems subjected to security assessment before deployment; penetration testing every 6 months; access control and audit logging verified; incident response

					plan includes AI-specific breach protocol; regulatory notification timelines (HIPAA 72hr, CERT-In 6hr) documented and assigned
Clinical Over-Reliance	Clinicians defer to AI recommendations without adequate critical evaluation, automation bias undermining independent clinical judgment	**3**	**4**	**12**	AI literacy training includes explicit automation bias module; documentation requirement when overriding AI recommendations; monthly review of override rate by department; culture of AI critical use modelled by senior clinicians
Vendor Failure	AI vendor ceases operations, is acquired, or is unable to maintain system performance, disrupting clinical workflows that have become dependent on AI	**2**	**4**	**8**	Multi-vendor strategy where possible; contractual data portability requirements; downtime procedures tested annually; escrow arrangement for AI model and training data; governance transition plan for vendor acquisition scenario
Staff Resistance Escalation	Organised resistance to AI adoption by clinical staff groups, creating	**2**	**3**	**6**	Proactive change management: staff involvement from design phase; champion

	implementation failure and institutional conflict				programme; transparent performance data sharing; clear escalation pathway for clinical concerns; leadership visible commitment to addressing legitimate concerns
Regulatory Non-Compliance	AI system use found to violate FDA, CDSCO, HIPAA, GDPR, or other applicable regulatory requirements, creating legal and reputational risk	**2**	**5**	**10**	Pre-deployment regulatory review by legal and compliance team; AI Ethics Committee includes legal representation; regulatory landscape monitoring programme; annual compliance audit of all live AI systems; regulatory breach response protocol documented
Patient Safety Incident	AI system recommendation contributes to patient harm, whether through incorrect output, misinterpretation, or failure to alert when alert was warranted	**2**	**5**	**10**	Formal AI adverse event reporting system parallel to clinical incident reporting; immediate suspension protocol for AI systems implicated in serious harm; root cause analysis required for all AI-related incidents;

					transparent reporting to Ethics Committee and board

Appendix D

Quality Metrics Dashboard

This dashboard provides a comprehensive quality measurement framework for an AI-integrated world-class hospital. Metrics are organised by domain with specific measurement methods, targets, and review cadence. The dashboard should be implemented in a digital quality management system with real-time data feeds from EHR and AI systems wherever possible.

DOMAIN 1: PATIENT SAFETY			
KPI / Metric	**Measurement Method**	**Target / Benchmark**	**Review Frequency**
Hospital-Acquired Infections			
CLABSI rate	Central line days and infections from infection surveillance system	<1.0 per 1,000 central line days (NHSN benchmark)	Monthly
CAUTI rate	Catheter days and UTIs from infection surveillance	<1.5 per 1,000 catheter days	Monthly
C. difficile rate	Laboratory confirmed CDI from infection control data	<0.5 per 10,000 patient days	Monthly
Hand hygiene compliance	Direct observation audits + AI-monitored dispenser usage	>90% compliance rate	Weekly
Medication Safety			

Medication error rate	Incident reports + BCMA override analysis from EHR	<0.5 errors per 100 medication administrations	Monthly
High-alert medication compliance	Barcode administration compliance rate from EHR	>99% barcode verification for high-alert medications	Weekly
Adverse drug event rate	Trigger tool review + incident reports	<5 ADEs per 1,000 patient days	Monthly
AI Safety Metrics			
Sepsis AI alert response rate	% alerts reviewed within 30 min from the EHR AI module	>85% reviewed within 30 minutes of alert generation	Daily
AI alert override rate	% AI recommendations overridden by clinicians	10–25% override rate (too low = automation bias; too high = alert fatigue)	Monthly
AI-related incidents	AI incident register, count and severity classification	Zero serious AI-related patient harm events	Monthly

DOMAIN 2: CLINICAL QUALITY AND EFFECTIVENESS			
KPI / Metric	**Measurement Method**	**Target / Benchmark**	**Review Frequency**
Sepsis Management			
Door-to-antibiotic time (sepsis)	EHR timestamp from sepsis alert to antibiotic administration	<60 minutes in >90% of sepsis cases	Monthly
Sepsis bundle compliance	AI-monitored bundle element documentation in EHR	>90% compliance with full Hour-1 Bundle	Monthly
Sepsis mortality	Sepsis deaths as % of sepsis diagnoses	Trend below the national average; year-on-year improvement	Quarterly
Surgical Quality			
Surgical site infection rate	SSI surveillance data by procedure category	<2% for clean-contaminated procedures	Monthly
Surgical Safety Checklist compliance	Direct audit + EHR documentation	>98% compliance (all three time-outs)	Weekly
Return to theatre rate (unplanned)	EHR procedure and complication data	<1% within 30 days of primary procedure	Monthly
Patient Experience			
Overall patient satisfaction	Structured patient survey (HCAHPS USA / NABH	>85th percentile national benchmark	Monthly

	equivalent India)		
Communication clarity rating	Patient survey, 'staff explained things clearly'	>90% 'always' response	Monthly
Compassion score	Validated patient experience tool (CARE Measure)	Mean score >45/50	Monthly

DOMAIN 3: OPERATIONAL EFFICIENCY AND AI PERFORMANCE			
KPI / Metric	**Measurement Method**	**Target / Benchmark**	**Review Frequency**
Operational Metrics			
Bed occupancy rate	Average beds occupied / total beds × 100 from the ADT system	80–85% (optimal range; above 90% = strain)	Daily
Average length of stay	EHR discharge data by diagnosis category vs. benchmark	Within 10% of the DRG/national benchmark	Monthly
ED wait time, door to physician	EHR timestamp from registration to physician contact	Median <30 min; 90th percentile <60 min	Daily
Operating theatre utilisation	Scheduled vs. actual OR utilisation from the scheduling system	>80% utilisation; <10% cancellation rate	Weekly
AI System Performance			
AI model sensitivity (by system)	Performance monitoring against the validation study baseline	Within 10% of validation study sensitivity	Monthly
AI model specificity (by system)	Performance monitoring against validation study baseline	Within 10% of validation study specificity	Monthly
Documentation burden reduction	Physician documentation time	>30% reduction in documentation	Quarterly

	before/after AI assistance	time per patient	
Alert fatigue rate	% AI alerts dismissed without review within required timeframe	<20% dismissal rate without review	Monthly

DOMAIN 4: WORKFORCE QUALITY AND DEVELOPMENT			
KPI / Metric	**Measurement Method**	**Target / Benchmark**	**Review Frequency**
Staff Competency and Training			
AI literacy training completion	LMS completion data, role-specific AI training	>95% completion by all staff within 6 months of deployment	Monthly
Clinical competency assessment	Direct observation, simulation assessment, Mini-CEX scores	>90% staff meeting competency threshold for key clinical skills	Quarterly
Quality improvement participation	Number of active QI projects per department	Minimum 1 active QI project per department at all times	Quarterly
Staff Wellbeing			
Staff burnout rate	Validated burnout tool (MBI or equivalent) administered annually	<20% high burnout prevalence across all clinical departments	Annual
Staff turnover rate	HR data, voluntary departures as % of total headcount	<15% annual turnover rate for clinical staff	Quarterly
Safety reporting rate	Near-miss and incident reports per 100 occupied bed days	Increasing rate year-on-year (reflects safety culture, not increasing harm)	Monthly

Appendix E

Training Programs for Staff and Students

This appendix provides the framework for the core training programmes required in a world-class AI-integrated healthcare institution. Each programme is defined by target audience, duration, content, delivery method, and assessment approach. All programmes should be reviewed annually and updated to reflect AI technology advances, regulatory changes, and local learning needs.

Programme	Audience	Duration	Core Content	Delivery Method	Assessment
AI Literacy Foundation	All clinical and administrative staff	4 hours (e-learning + workshop)	What AI is; how it works in healthcare; your role in AI governance; patient privacy and AI; how to use and critically evaluate AI recommendations in your role	Online modules + facilitated workshop with role-specific case discussions; peer-led delivery preferred	MCQ test >80%; signed acknowledgment of governance obligations
AI Clinical Champion Training	Designated AI champions, one per department	2 days intensive	In-depth AI performance metrics; alert calibration; troubleshooting AI integration issues; facilitating peer AI adoption; reporting governance concerns; change management skills	Intensive in-person programme; simulation exercises; champion competency assessment	Champion competency checklist; supervised facilitation of department AI training
AI Ethics and Governance	AI Ethics Committee members; department heads; senior	1 day workshop + quarterly updates	Bioethics principles applied to AI; bias auditing methodology; regulatory framework (FDA,	Workshop + case study analysis; regulatory update e-	Case study assessment; governance participation record

	clinical leaders		CDSCO, GDPR); AI Ethics Committee processes; incident management; annual governance report preparation	modules quarterly	
Lean Six Sigma Yellow Belt	All department staff, clinical and non-clinical	2 days	Waste identification (TIMWOODS); process mapping; basic problem-solving tools; PDCA cycle; how to participate in improvement projects and kaizen events	In-person workshop with local process improvement exercises	Improvement project participation; practical assessment
Lean Six Sigma Green Belt	Department improvement leads; charge nurses; quality coordinators	5 days + project	DMAIC methodology; statistical process control basics; value stream mapping; root cause analysis; project management for improvement; AI and quality integration	Classroom + supervised improvement project of measurable scope	Improvement project completion with documented outcomes; written assessment
Patient Safety and Quality	All new clinical staff (onboarding) + annual refresher	1 day initial; 2 hours annual	Swiss Cheese Model; error reporting culture; safety reporting system; incident investigation basics; patient safety national goals; your accountability for safety	In-person on onboarding; e-learning for annual refresher	Safety reporting system competency check; scenario-based assessment
Clinical Communication Skills	All clinical staff (doctors,	2 days + ongoing practice	SBAR for handover; breaking difficult	Facilitated workshop with SP	SP encounter assessment; 360-degree

	nurses, allied health)		news (SPIKES); shared decision-making; patient-centered consultation; telephone and telemedicine communication; AI disclosure language	encounters and video feedback; ongoing OSCE practice	feedback at 6 months
CBME AI Integration (Medical Students)	MBBS students, Years 1-4	Longitudinal across curriculum	Foundational AI literacy (Year 1); AI in clinical settings (Year 2); supervised AI use in clerkships (Year 3); AI governance and critical evaluation (Year 4); AI literacy teaching to peers (Year 4)	Integrated in clinical teaching, simulation, and ward rounds, not a standalone module	AI case analysis portfolio; OSCE AI scenario station; annual AI literacy assessment
Faculty AI Development	All teaching faculty	Tiered: Foundation (1 day), Intermediate (2 days), Advanced (3 days)	AI as clinical tool; AI as teaching tool; AI as subject to teach; facilitating AI critical discussions; assessing AI literacy in students; AI in curriculum design and CBME integration	Workshop + supervised AI-integrated teaching session observed by peers	Peer observation of AI-integrated teaching; faculty AI literacy assessment
Leadership AI Strategy	C-suite, board members, department heads	Half-day workshop + quarterly updates	AI governance framework; regulatory landscape (FDA/CDSCO/GDPR); AI Ethics Committee oversight; AI investment decision framework; AI risk management;	Executive workshop format; expert faculty; real case study discussions	Leadership commitment action plan; board AI governance participation

			leading AI culture change		

Appendix F

Role of Trustees

Trustees carry three fundamental legal and ethical duties:

1. Duty of Care

Act with the diligence of a reasonably prudent person, attend meetings, review materials, ask informed questions, and make thoughtful decisions

2. Duty of Loyalty

Place the institution's mission above personal, political, or business interests. Declare and recuse from any conflict of interest.

3. Duty of Obedience

Ensure the institution remains faithful to its stated charitable mission, quality healthcare and medical education for the community.

Specific Trustee Responsibilities

Strategic Direction

- Approve and periodically revise the institutional mission, vision, and strategic plan
- Set 3–5 year goals for hospital growth and academic program development

Financial Stewardship

- Approve annual budget and capital expenditure plans
- Review audited financial statements
- Ensure adequate reserves and financial sustainability
- Oversee fund utilization: grants, donations, government schemes (Ayushman Bharat, PMJAY)

Leadership Accountability

- Appoint, evaluate, and (if necessary) remove the Medical Superintendent and Principal/Dean
- Set performance expectations and compensation within non-profit guidelines

Compliance & Risk Oversight

- Ensure compliance with NMC (National Medical Commission) regulations
- Monitor NABH accreditation status
- Oversee legal, regulatory, and reputational risks

Mission Fulfillment

- Ensure the hospital provides equitable care, including free/subsidized services per trust deed obligations
- Protect the institution's charitable tax-exempt status (12A, 80G registrations)

What Trustees Should NOT Do

- Interfere in day-to-day clinical or administrative operations (that's management's role)
- Direct individual staff or departments without going through leadership
- Derive personal financial benefit from trust assets

Key Metrics & KPIs the Board Should Review

CLINICAL / HOSPITAL PERFORMANCE	
KPI	**Target Benchmark**
Bed Occupancy Rate (BOR)	70–85%
Average Length of Stay (ALOS)	Specialty-appropriate; track trend
OPD/IPD Patient Volume (monthly)	Month-over-month growth
Emergency Response Time	< 30 minutes for critical cases
Surgical Site Infection Rate	< 2%
Maternal Mortality Rate	Below district/state average
Patient Mortality Rate (adjusted)	Risk-adjusted, trended quarterly
Readmission Rate (30-day)	< 10%
Patient Satisfaction Score (NABH surveys)	> 85% satisfaction
Medical Error / Adverse Event Reports	Zero tolerance; full root-cause analysis

ACADEMIC / MEDICAL COLLEGE PERFORMANCE	
KPI	**Target Benchmark**
MBBS/PG Seat Utilization Rate	> 95% enrollment
NEXT / NEET-PG Pass Rate	≥ State average
Faculty-to-Student Ratio	NMC prescribed norms
Qualified Faculty Vacancy Rate	< 10%
Research Publications (annual)	Growing year-on-year
CME/Training Hours per Faculty	≥ 30 hrs/year
NMC Inspection Compliance Score	Full compliance
Student Feedback Score	> 80% positive

World Class Healthcare & Medical Education, By Jay P. Patel I Quality & Productivity Solutions, Inc. I www.qpsinc.com

AI +Digital TRaansformation + Quality + Leadership +Human Values = Better Healthcare

WHAT DOES WORLD-CLASS HEALTHCARE LOOK LIKE?

Healthcare is not just another industry. It is about human life, dignity, and trust. And it stands today at a moment of historic transformation, one in which artificial intelligence, applied with discipline, wisdom, and genuine human values, can extend world-class care to patients who have never had access to it.

WHAT YOU WILL FIND INSIDE

- **AI Implementation RoadMap** the four-phase framework from awareness through scale, for every hospital, in every context
- **World-Class Physician Criteria** seven measurable competencies including soft skills, leadership, and human-centered thinking, with global benchmarks from Johns Hopkins, CMC Vellore, AIIMS, Karolinska, and Harvard
- **USA and India Relationship**, FDA, NABH, GDPR, the EU AI Act, and NMC, what every leader must know and do

- **Quality + AI Integration** Lean Six Sigma applied to healthcare, the DMAIC framework, and the quality-driven AI system
- **Five Ready-to-Use Appendices** AI Implementation Checklist, Hospital Readiness Assessment, Risk Register, Quality Metrics Dashboard, and Training Programs

Written for every leader and professional

Hospital administrators | Medical directors | Faculty and educators | Policymakers | Medical students

With the right knowledge, discipline, and values, transformation is always possible. This is where it begins.

ABOUT THE AUTHOR

Jay P. Patel is a leader, quality Fellow, educator and international consultant with over 30 years of experience transforming organizations across manufacturing, technology, and healthcare globally. He holds a Master's degree and MBA from universities in the United States. He has authored 10+ books, 10 more books are in process.

He is the founder and CEO of Quality & Productivity Solutions, Inc. and the visionary leader.

Technology empowers.
Quality ensures excellence.
Humanity remains at the center.

www.ingramcontent.com/pod-product-compliance
Lightning Source LLC
LaVergne TN
LVHW071412210926
848486LV00004B/254